Pullingthe**trigger**®

There is recovery and a place beyond. We promise.

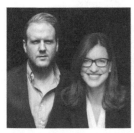 Adam Shaw, a mental illness survivor and mental health advocate, and Lauren Callaghan, an industry-leading clinical psychologist, are the founders of the global mental health publishing enterprise, **Pulling**the**trigger**®. With their TV appearances and global education programmes, Adam, Lauren and their amazing team are helping more people around the world understand, recover from, and talk about their mental health issues.

The **Pulling**the**trigger**® range – user-friendly self-help books with an innovative approach to supporting people recovering from mental health issues.

The**inspirational**series™ – remarkable, real-life stories of men and women who have overcome mental illness to lead fulfilling lives.

Why have we called our books Pulling the**trigger**®?

Many things can 'trigger' mental health issues. So what do you do if something makes you feel bad? You stay away from it, right?

I bet you've been avoiding your triggers all your life. But now we know that avoiding them only makes things worse. So here's the game changer: you need to learn how to pull those triggers instead of running away from them – and our **Pulling**the**trigger**® series shows you how. Your recovery is within reach, we promise.

This is more than recovery, it's a way of life.

Adam Shaw & Lauren Callaghan.

First published in Great Britain 2017 by Trigger Press

Trigger Press is a trading style of Shaw Callaghan Ltd & Shaw Callaghan 23 USA, INC.

The Foundation Centre
Navigation House, 48 Millgate, Newark
Nottinghamshire NG24 4TS UK

www.trigger-press.com

British Library Cataloguing in Publication Data

A CIP catalogue record for this book is available upon request
from the British Library

ISBN: 978-1-911246-45-9

This book is also available in the following e-Book formats:

MOBI: 978-1-911246-48-0
EPUB: 978-1-911246-46-6
PDF: 978-1-911246-47-3

Cover design and typeset by Fusion Graphic Design Ltd

Project Management by Out of House Publishing

Printed and bound in Great Britain by Bell & Bain, Glasgow

Paper from responsible sources

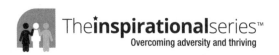

The**inspirational**series™
Overcoming adversity and thriving

Shiny Happy Person
Finding the Sun Between Clouds of Depression
By Terri Cox

We are proud to introduce The**inspirational**series™. Part of the **Pulling**the**trigger**® family of innovative self-help mental health books, The**inspirational**series™ tells the stories of the people who have battled and beaten mental health issues. For more information visit: www.pulling-the-trigger.com

THE AUTHOR

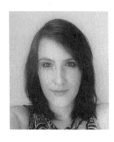

Terri Cox suffered with undiagnosed depression and anxiety in her early twenties before having a mental breakdown in 2015. With the help of her family, friends and psychotherapist, she managed to pull herself out of the dark pit of despair and is now passionate about sharing her story and awareness of mental health in any way that she can.

Terri now lives in Hull, where she has a dream job using her European languages skills. She enjoys needlecraft, comedy sitcoms and travelling around the UK.

Thank you for purchasing this book.
You are making an incredible difference.

All of The**inspirational**series™ products have substantial
enterprising and philanthropic value and generate proceeds that
contribute towards our global mental health charity,
The Shaw Mind Foundation

MISSION STATEMENT

*'We aim to bring to an end the suffering and despair caused
by mental health issues. Our goal is to make help and support
available for every single person in society, from all walks of life.
We will never stop offering hope. These are our promises.'*

Pulling the Trigger and The Shaw Mind Foundation

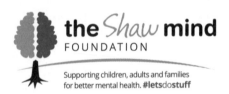

The Shaw Mind Foundation (www.shawmindfoundation.org) offers
unconditional support for all who are affected by mental health
issues. We are a global foundation that is not for profit. Our core
ethos is to help those with mental health issues and their families at
the point of need. We also continue to run and invest in mental health
treatment approaches in local communities around the globe, which
support those from the most vulnerable and socially deprived areas
of society. Please join us and help us make an incredible difference
to those who are suffering with mental health issues. **#lets**do**stuff**.

To all my superheroes.

Disclaimer: Some names and identifying details have been changed to protect the privacy of individuals.

PROLOGUE

It's Saturday August 17th, 2013, about 9.00pm. I'm in a Wetherspoon's pub on a night out that I've been looking forward to for a good few weeks. It's the weekend after my 23rd birthday, and I am going to celebrate by dancing, laughing too much, and enjoying the sweet chemical taste of cheap drinks. My friends have gathered; I'm wearing a pretty black jump suit with yellow flowers. To me, it's beautiful. I've just lost three stone and even though I will eventually have to lose another three, I still feel like hot stuff. The jump suit was a lucky accidental find, and having been taken in by vanity sizing, I'm sporting a size 14. The matching shoes only took a six-hour shopping trip to find.

I pop to the bar. Hordes of 'twenty-somethings' cram in like sardines to get in on the 2-for-£10 cocktail pitcher deal. I buy a questionable drink that's meant to be like an alcoholic Vimto. I pay, pick up my pitcher, turn in my tracks, and take a few steps forward towards the throng.

Here's what this moment reminds me of. In the Harry Potter books (yes, I'm one of those devout fans) there is a moment where Harry is rapped on the head with someone's wand, in order to be turned invisible. A strange feeling spreads downwards as if someone has smashed an egg on his head and it's running down his body. Only for me, the feeling is nasty and cold. It's a feeling that goes to my chest, grips my heart and stops me in my tracks for a couple of seconds. Brief, but paralysing.

An overwhelming feeling of 'what is the point?' descends.

It disappears almost as soon as it appears. But I am left with a sense of confusion that lingers for days.

CHAPTER 1

BEGIN THE BEGIN

In most ways, I'm a normal woman. My name is Terri and at the time of writing, I am 26-years-old. I have a boyfriend and a job I enjoy. I have friends and a family that I love, and I live in a great little flat.

So why am I writing a book? And why should it be of any interest to anyone?

The simple answer is: I'm writing this because I am normal. I have suffered with depression, and that's normal. Mental illness isn't okay but, unfortunately, it is common.

Just as there are thousands of illnesses and diseases that exist in the human body, so there are several illnesses of the mind. 1 in 6 people suffered from mental health in the last week[1]. We shouldn't be surprised about this. Given what I've been through, I shouldn't be surprised by it. But I am.

The problem is that mental illness is frequently invisible. As my mother always says to me – you can see a broken arm, it can't be hidden. If you see someone bruised and bloodied after falling in the street, you rush to help them. If somebody walks in with their arm in a cast, you immediately sympathise and ask how they are. But you can't always see the effects of a poorly mind.

1 www.mentalhealth.org.uk/statistics/mental-health-statistics-uk-and-worldwide

Before I had one, I didn't even know what a breakdown was. It was something I occasionally heard about if there was someone brave enough to tell me they'd had one, but honestly, nobody had ever described it to me in detail. And I didn't ask for details. It's not the accepted etiquette to ask someone why they had a breakdown. It's not seen as polite. But I wouldn't think twice about asking somebody how they broke a bone. I would even laugh along with them when they told me their exaggerated story of how it happened.

The truth is, it's hard to empathise with somebody about something that you have never experienced, and even harder when it's not socially accepted to talk about it in detail.

There's a lot about mental illness that I know and understand nothing about. Maybe I'll learn more as I go along, maybe from other books like this one. For now, though, what follows is a personal account.

When I had low-level depression, I could still prioritise the feelings of other people. I could even still help – sometimes to the detriment of dealing with my own issues. However, when the situation steadily declined and I ultimately fell into a breakdown, I wasn't capable of that anymore. By their nature, depression and anxiety have the potential to strip away your ability to consider the personal struggles of anyone around you. I don't mean to say that it makes you a selfish or a bad person – I just mean that it can render you unable to consider the possibility that you aren't the only one suffering. And that makes it an even lonelier place to be.

Let it be known that there were people in my life that were having their own battles with mental illness alongside me in this timeline. However, I can't, and wouldn't want to, tell their story for them. I can only share what happened to me.

I am writing for the people that are currently suffering and need hope. I am writing for their families, who maybe can't understand and just want some guidance to help them through the fear. I'm writing for my family, because even those who have been there for most of it still won't understand the full picture. I'm hoping, after reading it, people will feel okay asking me questions. Lots of questions. I don't mind. Sometimes it's easier to answer than to volunteer the information.

If you think you see or know anyone going through any of the things that you read here, please tell them that they're normal. Tell them it can change. Tell them that they don't have to keep it secret if they feel they need to get it out somehow. Tell them you'll be there for them.

The more we can talk about it, the more normal it becomes. We can shine a beaming spotlight on the evil disease that hides in the shadows and expose it for what it really is. And the more people we can help.

CHAPTER 2

WHEN I WAS YOUNG

I was born in 1990 to David and Julie in Hull, England, as one of a set of identical triplets. My parents already had two daughters – Natalie aged eight, and Nicola aged nine. They already had two 'T' names lined up, Toni and Terri, but couldn't think of a third. They asked the nurses at the hospital to name the third baby, and they came up with Stephanie.

We were studious children, with an addiction to reading. Dad would bring home reams of paper that were used at his job as a fish filleter, and he would cut it up into hundreds of individual squares. We wrote tons of stories and illustrated them. I remember that we thought we could only stick to the one sheet of paper, and so we would squash our writing as small as possible at the bottom of the page to fit it all on.

We all loved primary school. So many happy memories ... We sang hymns that we still remember to this day. We loved the book fair that would pop up a couple of times a year, scouring the catalogues and choosing a brightly coloured book. We always chose fiction. We remember our primary school head teacher, Mr Ibson. He was a smiley, friendly man who made the school a fun and happy place to be. Sometimes, if I smell apple pie or acrylic paints, I'm immediately transported back to those classrooms.

We loved anything to do with crafts – everything from designing the Christmas decorations for our class display to building small wooden cars and kites to race with the other kids. If we were creating something, we threw ourselves into it.

We shared our pocket money and bought all of the same book series, signing every cover with 'This book belongs to Toni, Terri, and Stephanie Cox.' I remember our parents telling friends that the three of us were absolutely obsessed with reading. If Mam told us that we were banned from reading books or magazines at the table so that we could concentrate on our food, we would resort to reading the back of the cereal boxes or condiments instead. While we brushed our teeth, we would read the back of the shampoo bottles. Dad told us that we were like his mother, who we'd never had a chance to meet – she loved reading too.

Our older sister, Natalie, was a home-bird and could lie in for longer than anyone I had ever met. I remember the times when we couldn't sleep and she'd pop her head around the bedroom door, singing funny songs to make us laugh or telling us about Father Christmas.

Nikki lived with our grandma for a couple of years, just a couple of streets away from us. And when Grandma would babysit for us, we would sleep in Nikki's room. I remember thinking she was so cool because she had pictures of boybands on her walls and glow-in-the-dark stickers on her bedroom ceiling. She would tickle us and make us laugh until we cried. When we were 10, Nikki had a baby boy – our first nephew, Kai – and they came to live with us. He was a beautiful baby. Sometimes, on our way home from school, Toni, Steph and I would argue about who got to give Kai a bath when we got home.

As I came to high school age, I was disappointed that Nat and Nikki had already left school. Would it have made a difference to our experience if they'd still been there? They both said they wished they'd been there to look after us.

Our parents divorced when we were 11-years-old. Dad moved out but continued to live close by, so we were still able to see him really often. It wasn't a clean divorce. There was a lot of animosity between them. Fortunately, we were too young to know the details, and quite frankly, I didn't want to know. It hurt too much.

I don't remember how long it took, or what sparked it, but eventually they stopped speaking face-to-face. Things were just too difficult for them to keep talking to each other. Even phone calls and text messages were out of the question. Communication, when it absolutely had to happen, was through handwritten notes. While that spared our parents having to speak to each other, it didn't spare us from watching or hearing their reactions.

I was worried about it all the time. When we were alone, Toni, Steph, and I would argue about who had to hand the next note over. When I knew I was going to Mam or Dad's house the next day, I would spend the whole night worrying, sometimes dreaming about handing the note over. I got way past the point of ever wishing for parents who would get back together, or even parents who would be friends. I just didn't want things to carry on like that.

Mam got remarried to Stan a couple of years later. I don't remember making it very easy for them for a long time. I was a demon child at that point! A teenage girl naturally clashes with her mother anyway, but I was struggling badly. I was always argumentative and snapped and shouted at everyone around me. From reading my diaries, I know that I was utterly miserable: worried at home, stressed with my sisters, and terrified at school.

A lot of people ask if I have a psychic connection to my triplet sisters, or if we can read each other's minds. As much as I laugh along with the jokes, I don't believe in any of that. But, to prove how much we lived in each other's pockets, there are a handful of memories the three of us share that we all claim as our own. There was the winter's day on the school run where the pavement was slick with ice and I couldn't stand up, slipping over every time I tried. Some of the other parents were trying to pick me up, but were struggling to keep their balance too. Toni and Stephanie are both *convinced*, beyond a shadow of a doubt, that it was them who experienced it. We haven't come to a conclusion about it in 20 years, and I don't think we ever will.

The three of us always argued, bickered, and even sometimes fought, all the way through our lives. At the point of high school, it was unbearable. Especially for those around us. Our family were pulling their hair out, and our friends were completely fed up.

We didn't stop arguing for long enough to consider what it must have been like for other people to be around. We bickered so much that nobody had time to stop and hear themselves think, never mind consider our point of view. So here is our point of view. This is the reality of living as one of three ...

I spent every waking minute with Toni and Stephanie. Not only did we obviously live together, but we shared the same room. We woke up together, ate breakfast together, travelled to school together, and because we were in the highest classes, we spent every single lesson together, where obviously we sat together too. Break times would be together because we had the same friends. We would travel home together, eat our evening meal together. We would go on holiday together, sleep at Grandma's house together. We would fight over time on the shared computer, shared TV, shared bedroom space. We would share birthday cards and gifts from certain family and friends. We would even share names. I would even have to answer to 'Toni' or 'Steph' from people speaking directly at me, because people would get it wrong. By high school, the teachers that had the most respect for us called us all Miss Cox. They had tried their hardest to learn our names, but it was too confusing for some of them. The other children that weren't our friends simply called us 'triplet'. I hated that. Only two people were allowed to call us 'trips', and that was our big sisters. It was affectionate coming from them, instead of rude.

Annoying, isn't it, how many times the word 'together' and 'shared' crops up in that paragraph?

Now, imagine living it. For years.

I loved Toni and Steph, and still love them more than anything in the world. Every single new experience, new challenge, new battle, new adventure that comes with growing up, we went through it at exactly the same time. And that may even continue in our adult lives.

Yes, there will have been a lot of things that were easier for me growing up than for people who didn't have that kind of relationship. When starting a new school, for example, I didn't ever have to worry about having nobody to speak to.

There were other benefits too. Every weekend we would pool together our pocket money and buy a new season of *Friends*, a new film, a new set of books or a new CD, knowing full well that normally it would have taken us weeks to save up for them ourselves. We had the same hobbies and exactly the same sense of humour. I still laugh when I remember the giggling fits the three of us would get into when somebody said something funny in class – the fact that no one else found it amusing made it even funnier.

As strange as it may sound to anyone who hasn't experienced it, our whole identities were defined by who we were as a three, right up until we left school. You know all those times as a child or a teen when you got to hang out by yourself in your room and shut off the rest of the world, or go out with a friend that was just yours, or have a day out without your family? None of that was possible for us.

We also studied the exact same subjects, so the jealousy was hard to handle when one of us received an award that the others didn't. *Why did she get it when I didn't?* we'd ask ourselves. *What's wrong with me?*

It's hard to listen to people telling you not to compare yourself to your sisters when you are supposed to be literally the same in every way. It's even harder when you're constantly compared to each other by everyone who knows your family or stops you in the street.

In the next chapter, I'll talk about some of the things we experienced in school that made all three of us absolutely miserable. Every single kid in the school knew who we were, even if we didn't have a clue who they were. Bullying was a sport. A spectator sport. I think in the times we are living in, to some extent that's true in most schools. It was even more amusing to our persecutors, because we were triplets. It was a sport they could all join in on.

As a three, it was a terrifying, stressful, devastating, and confusing time. We were so angry. We believed that these things wouldn't be happening to us if we weren't triplets. We were geeky, gawky, bespectacled, taller than every other kid, and chubby. And because it was all multiplied by three, we stuck out like three sore thumbs. But we had more safety in numbers, and so we were terrified to leave each other's sides. We felt like magnets; we would stick fast to each other because it was natural, but we also felt trapped and unable to ever get away because we had no other options.

My therapist has since described it as being like a jar of bees. When you're trapped in an environment with such little freedom, the energy still has to go somewhere. The anger, the bitterness, the stress, and especially the blame, just had to go somewhere. We took it out on each other and everyone around us felt the shockwaves. Over and over again, people screamed at us that we just enjoyed the arguing. No matter how many times we said we didn't, what reason did they have to believe us? We were arguing non-stop. If you don't want to argue, just don't argue. How simple is that?

We can't 'break up' the way an arguing couple would. And I wouldn't want them to be gone from my life. I love them too much.

A year ago, we found ourselves a joint counsellor to help us resolve the disputes that still continue. She is currently helping undo all the damage that's been done over the years, all the ways we learned to communicate with each other using nastiness and shouting. It's therapeutic and we'll continue to work on it for as long as it takes to break such a bloody miserable long-term habit.

As things are now, we have separate lives. Throughout higher education and after, we have had different levels of involvement in each other's lives. Now, my sisters are successful women in jobs that they really enjoy, as am I. We all live and work in different cities, but I still speak to them all day, every day. We call, text, and email.

The independence is freeing, but we still want to hear from each other, and when something goes wrong, that magnet pull is still there. They are the first people I send a message to at the end of a stressful day, the first people I run to for help, and the first people I will inform of anything big that happens in my life.

Now, when they achieve something great, I celebrate it instead of feeling jealous. I'm so proud of them. That will always be true no matter how hard it may be for outsiders to believe.

My family. I love them more than I can say. They're all a large part of this whole story and a big part of how I came so far.

CHAPTER 3

BAD DAY

I would be here for a very long time if I were to write out all my memories of bullying. But there are a few that stand out the most. I call one of them Lights Out.

Halfway through my time at high school, a new building was built on the site of the upper school. Modern. Bright colours.

I hated those bright colours. They were a complete lie. Look at this lovely school we have here. What a haven! Everything is bright and happy and children go skipping down the corridors singing, hand-in-hand.

Some kids must have worked out what time my sisters and I had our English class down one of those corridors. A couple of minutes before the class ended, two kids had stationed themselves at either end of the corridor, and simultaneously turned out the lights when they saw us leave the classroom. I felt a swift kick to my ankle and I hit the deck, at which point they got in a few extra kicks to the face, gut, and legs for good measure. When the lights came back on, I had no idea who had beaten me up.

Some of the teachers would do anything to help us. We had a physics teacher who we adored. We approached him, upset, after a particularly nasty class, and explained what had been happening to us in his lesson. He was enraged. He lined everybody up along the back wall, and he didn't mention names. He paced the classroom, explaining how bullies were scum and if he were to ever, ever hear that any bullying had gone on in his class again, he would make sure each of them was marched directly to the headmistress to be dealt with, and he would personally call their parents. It didn't happen again for as long as I was in his class.

Some of the teachers would do nothing to help us, no matter what happened. One year we had a maths class in which we were using compasses and protractors to cut shapes out of card, which we'd then assemble into 3D geometric shapes. I'll never forget the sight of Stephanie crying in pain from compasses being thrown at her back and head. Our friends Sarah, Laura, and Sam grabbed as many of the shapes those kids had made as possible, and crushed them in rage.

I'll leave you to guess who was told off.

My father was fuming. Parents' evening was approaching and he asked to go instead of my mother for this particular session. When we arrived at the school, he made a beeline straight for the maths teacher.

'I have a question for you. Why did you become a teacher?'

She stammered, confused. 'Sorry?'

'My girls are being bullied in your class. Some of the boys in your class are throwing sharp things at them. It's *dangerous*, and when you were told about it, you got mad at them for ripping up some of their work.'

'I understand that they were upset, but no matter what happens I can't condone pupils destroying each other's work. A lot of effort had gone into it.'

'But you can ignore violence? I don't give a knack about a bit of cardboard. If they're going to hurt my daughters then I don't blame them. They're scared to go into your class. You're a teacher and it's your job to deal with it. I want to know what you're going to do about it.'

'The problem is—'

'No! I don't want to hear it. What are you going to do about it?'

'What you need to understand is—'

'You aren't listening to me. What are you going to do about it? Do I have to go to your bosses?'

'With disturbed children like those, you have to make special allowances for them.'

Dad was stunned into silence for a few seconds. But then he spoke again.

'So what you mean is, you have to go easy on them and let them get away with it because it's too hard to deal with them properly? In the meantime, they're throwing compasses at my daughters.'

All of these things were horrible to experience. The fear of something happening to you every minute of every day was exhausting. But no matter how scared I was for myself, it didn't compare to the fear I had whenever I saw something happening to my sisters. I would have taken their place in a heartbeat.

One day, on the way to science class, I was walking along with my friends and my sisters were walking side-by-side a couple of paces behind. Suddenly I heard a ruckus behind me. I turned around and saw Toni cowering in tears while a much older girl punched her face and the top of her head with all her might. The mixture of fear, shock, pain, and hurt on her face was mirrored by the white ball of panic and fury in my chest. And I just stood there, terrified.

I don't remember the exact details, but somehow a few seconds later, the three of us were standing in a nearby classroom with a teacher. It transpired that the girl wasn't even a pupil from our school. She was the cousin of a girl in our class that had tried to hit one of us and been mortally offended when Toni had fought back to stop her. This girl was an absolute nutcase, much older than us. I genuinely believe it was nothing but a coincidence that she had managed to choose Toni out of the three of us to 'get her own back'.

Toni was bright red and crying, and that's when my tears came out. I was devastated, but I couldn't contain the guilt I felt from being frozen to the spot and not jumping in to stop it happening. Steph was hugging her tightly and I just couldn't do anything except stand and sob and say I was sorry over and over again.

Yes, the place was a shithole. But weren't they all? I *hate* to think how many people had similar experiences. There will be hundreds upon thousands of similar stories left untold. How many children, like us, were pounded with snowballs that were packed with rocks or razorblades? How many had to walk into their school toilets to find insulting and disgusting comments about them written in giant writing across the wall?

I remember my mother getting out of her car once when she was picking us up from school, and running towards a bus stop where she saw one child being attacked by two others. She was shaking and almost crying when she got back into the car, and called the school to let them know. It can't have been easy for her to actually see the kind of thing her daughters and their friends were going through themselves.

I had long hair in high school. One day, I went to school with my hair in a braid. By mid-afternoon, my hair was wrapped in a girl's hand while she tried to set it alight with her lighter. She had insulted me for not being a smoker and I'd had had the nerve to talk back. That moment of fear is etched as clear as day on my mind, but no matter how hard I think about it, I can't remember how I got out of it.

There were also moments of comedy. For one, that uniform. Pure cruelty. Aubergine purple (or dish-water brown and bruise-purple jumpers for the unlucky kids who had managed to land themselves with a bad dye-lot).

By no means did we stay silent while we endured a torrent of verbal abuse. We were smart kids and annoying with it. We loved pointing out how stupid those kids were. We took every opportunity to pull apart whatever they said and make them look idiotic and moronic. Sarcasm was my favourite weapon.

They didn't like it. It was like throwing fuel on a fire. How *dare* we speak back? I cannot convey how many times somebody demanded to know to whom I believed I was talking.

'Oo you talking to, you?'

One day a girl took one look at the pinstripes that I was wearing on my trousers and demanded to know why I wasn't following the proper uniform rules, which called for plain black ones. In hindsight, I had two options. Shut the hell up and hope it blew over quicker. Or answer back.

I chose the latter. I took one long sarcastic look at her half-mast tracksuit bottom, tucked into her white socks and scruffy trainers, and told her she could call the cast of *Shameless* her rich, classy cousins. The punch that I got to the face was almost, *almost* worth the few seconds of slack-jawed non-comprehension on her face before she realised that I had insulted her.

There were lots of times that my friends got their own back in ways that still make me laugh to this day; they help me cope with remembering what a shithole the place really was.

Our friend, Sam, was bullied worse than we were. I've never seen anyone else be so strong in the face of constant verbal and physical abuse. I saw her get kicked down an entire flight of stairs. I saw her being hit with metal poles. A thousand times a day she was called every name under the sun.

She showed up to the school every single day. She did not let the bastards win. She wasn't afraid of her own shadow; she would keep her voice loud above the crowd and didn't take anything lying down. She fought back when someone attacked her. She didn't show them tears.

Have you read *Matilda*? Or seen the film? It's about a young girl with powers who has terrible parents. She attends a school with an awful principal who has some very cruel, very theatrical methods of punishing any children who cross her. The principal used to be a heavyweight lifter and was a hammer throw expert. There is a moment when a small girl with pigtails makes her angry. In the school playground, the principal grabs the girl by her pigtails, swings her around in the air hammer throw style, and launches her right over the school gates onto the grass beyond.

Between the upper school and the lower school sites, there was a long stretch of grass where we used to run cross-country laps. (Well, some people ran, I resembled that lame rhinoceros at the end of the stampede in *Jumanji*). It was divided along the middle by one long gravel pathway. Whenever it rained for a significant period of time, the grass on either side would get flooded and transform into a swamp, complete with swarms of flies and an insane amount of mud – a lot of which would be flung in our direction fairly regularly.

A boy from school in the year above ours, in all his bravery, used to terrorise us younger girls weekly – always with a small army of other older boys behind him. (A true warrior!) He would steal the food we made in food technology class. He would trip us up and he would spit on us. One day he approached Sam and, using all the might of his Neanderthal brain, came up with an oh-so-original insult about her weight. When she replied with a quip instead of cowering in fear, the caveman became angry. He began to push her around.

I looked over at exactly the right time. Something snapped in Sam's eyes, and I saw her reach for the boy's backpack. He tried to keep hold of it, but with pure anger, she wrenched it from his grip. I have never seen such a beautiful throw. She spun on the spot, exactly like the principal in *Matilda*, and launched the bag through the air for an impressive distance, where it subsequently landed in the disgusting, muddy swampy water.

That was one of those times that Toni, Steph, and I had one of our giggling fits that made life in that place bearable.

CHAPTER 4

FINAL STRAW

By the age of 14, low self-esteem and mild anxiety were already a normal part of our lives. I was keeping a daily diary and I would pore over it for hours. I decorated it with cuttings from the hundreds of magazines I read. I still loved reading, and always would. But I think it was becoming less and less about just wanting to read a nice story, and more and more about keeping my mind busy and distracted.

Sundays were almost unbearable. There was a TV show that my mother would watch every Sunday evening called *Heartbeat*. The theme tune was insanely catchy. It came on every Sunday night at eight o'clock. The problem was that, after a while, I started to associate that tune with the Sunday night feeling. It was so much worse than that feeling of knowing I had to get up early and go to class the next day; it was the promise of a new week, and a whole new world of potential crap raining down on us. I was scared all the time about what was going to happen. If I hear that *Heartbeat* tune now, I still get anxious and have to fight the urge to kick a sheep!

I only have to look at my diary to see that by this time my self-esteem had been ripped to shreds:

You know what is really starting to annoy me? For the past couple of weeks, I've been getting this feeling of dread every time someone gives me a task to do. As soon as I look at a question, or have to draw or write something, I just start saying, 'I can't do it. I CAN'T DO IT!' over and over again.

I refused toast today as I pictured what I looked like in that white top. I really need to lose about two elephant's worth of weight, and probably even then some more.

Who wants to look like this in a prom dress? My goal is to look OK in a dress but right now I look like a swollen, overweight, pregnant, unusually large mammoth. How can anyone bear to look at me when I am so fat? I wish it could be like it was when I was little and I didn't care about being so fat – which I always have been, I know that.

I know very well that this low self-confidence didn't come from my home life. Our parents were constantly telling us how smart we were and how capable we were. They always called us pretty, beautiful, and told us to stop being so hard on ourselves.

In September 2004, we also experienced our first bereavement when we lost our grandma. I wrote about that too.

Mam was acting really strangely at breakfast. We sat and had a long talk about all sorts of things, and then she started saying, 'I don't understand it, I'm going to my mother's funeral tomorrow. I'm going to my mother's funeral. How do you get your head around that?' And then she said she felt guilty because somebody she knows had told her off for feeling sad and said that she had to 'think of the kids'. I told her that she'd been excellent considering what she was going through. Then she hugged me for a really long time and she was saying in my ear that we were the best things in her life, her five daughters.

A death in the family is a confusing and overwhelming experience for any child. School should have been a distraction, but I couldn't even relax then. Bullying, worries about my weight, and anxiety over my schoolwork were all still there underneath the grief.

When I go back to my diary, my head spins from reading it. I just want to go back in time and hug the poor young teen who just didn't know which emotion to deal with first.

I had a cry in Tutor Period today, and having a cry kind of helped the queasy feeling I had inside from trying not to cry for a couple of days. I had two biscuits for breakfast this morning because Mam wouldn't let me go to school without something to eat first. Miss wanted to send me home but I already have to miss school on Friday for the funeral and I can't afford to skip time, or I can't do my mock exams. I am so sick of worrying about what's going to happen every single break time, and lunch time and home time because of the bullying from the boys. It's so tiring.

Halfway through Year 10, when we were 14-years-old, we reached the tipping point.

It was morning break-time. Toni, Stephanie, and I were with our friends in the usual corner of the playground. It was partially behind a corner, where two buildings met, so we were safely tucked away from the masses. A boy came up behind Toni to hit her. As a reflex, Stephanie kicked out, just at the same moment as Toni pulled him off her, right into the path of Stephanie's foot. I heard the impact of her foot on his cheek ...

It can't have caused more than a bruise, but the fury and curses that came our way were horrible. He left with his friends in tow. It was an unpleasant few moments, but we tried to brush off the embarrassment.

The bell rang out and we made our way with our friends back to class, our friends reassuring us the whole way. But we had relaxed too soon. As we turned the corner a white mist filled the air, and when I stopped flinching I looked up to see my sister standing in the middle of the corridor, covered head to foot in flour. The boy had gone to the food department, taken somebody's casserole cornflour, and poured the whole bag over Stephanie's head.

There is an argument to be made that sometimes, fear, humiliation, and anxiety are worse than actual pain. My sisters were mortified and I was terrified. We were now guaranteed, at the very least, a whole day of ridicule from our class peers. I would have taken a quick punch to the face to be in her place at that moment. We cleaned her off the best we could. I tried to ignore my thumping heart and burning cheeks and eyes for the rest of the morning.

What happened next is known by our family as 'The Witch Hunt'. I can still use that term now, years later, and my family instantly know what I'm talking about.

Lunchtime came. Our school was a couple of streets away from home, so we would go home every day for cucumber sandwiches. (No, really!) We stepped out of the school and into the playground. It was a bit busier than usual directly outside the building, and so we prepped ourselves for walking closer together and faster, keeping our heads down. I didn't really know what was happening until I heard somebody ask one of my sisters which one of us had kicked the boy earlier.

When I looked up, my stomach lurched. There were dozens upon dozens of kids in a crowd all around us – bricks, wooden planks, stones all in hand. They had come to get us in one large group.

That long gravel pathway between the two schools never looked longer. The whole way to the lower school, we were pulled at, kicked, pushed, punched, hit with debris, soaked in drinks, spit, and sworn at.

'Look at the fat cow crying!' someone yelled, followed by nasty laughter.

A couple of our friends ran off back towards the school to tell the teachers what was happening. The rest of them flanked us. I kept my eyes forward and didn't dare look back, but at one point my sisters were ahead of me and both turned around to check where I was at the same time. The looks of sheer panic and the yelps of fear they both gave out will never leave my mind.

A passer-by yelled, but I didn't hear what they said. We just kept shouting at each other to keep moving.

We lived a five-minute walk away from the school. When we arrived home, we phoned our mother. Her voice shook as she talked to us down the line.

'Do *not* go back into school,' she told us. 'I'll be home as soon as I can, okay, darling? Stay where you are. It's going to be okay.'

She rushed home and called the school straightaway. The passer-by had called the school to report what they had seen.

We cried for the rest of the afternoon and my stomach was in pain from sobbing. Mam hugged us and swore in anger. She cried and promised to protect us. She made us a cup of tea each and told us to get settled down for the night.

We didn't return to school for two weeks after that. It was snowing anyway, and so we used that as a flimsy back-up reason for not going back in.

What is almost even more insulting than being beaten up or terrorised every day, is reaching out to people who have the authority to step in, to help, to support you and put an end to it all ... and they just don't. One evening, Mam drove us into school after hours and we had a meeting with the Head of Year. It was the bravest I have ever felt speaking my mind to a teacher. What was there to lose in being honest? There was no way they could punish me for being hurt. I was here with my mother and she was the only one in the room there who had any real intention of protecting us.

We told him that this had been going on the whole time we were there and that we were sick of not being listened to. At first, he told us that we were overreacting to a bit of teasing. (I think teachers with this attitude can be just as dangerous as the children actually doing the bullying.) We protested in outrage and my mother told him exactly what she thought of that.

The usual spiel followed. They had an *anti-bullying policy*. They took the incident *very seriously*. They were looking into talking to students to try to find out who had instigated it. In the meantime, we had already discussed at home the option of moving to another school. Two of us wanted to leave, but Toni wanted to stay. She was scared that if we went somewhere else, we could get even worse treatment. But at least here we knew what we were facing, and we had some friends. Besides, our GCSEs were coming up, and it was really important to all of us, but mostly Toni, that our grades weren't messed up. It made complete sense in that regard.

You would think that two out of three would win, but we would not force Toni to do something she didn't want to do, and we weren't going to be separated or leave her behind, alone.

The school came up with one hell of a strategy. What do you do when you have dozens of kids bullying three people? Do you punish the dozens of kids? Suspend them? Put them all in detention? No. You remove the victims from their reach.

This was the plan. Every morning, a teacher would collect us from home in their car. It was no trouble – we lived near the school and so it wasn't out of their way. We would arrive at school an hour earlier than all the other children. We would be dropped off at the back of the school where the door had been unlocked earlier that morning by the caretaker. We would walk through the empty, dark corridors and up to the library. We would close and lock the door behind us.

For a long time, we had to be escorted between classes by whichever teacher had just finished their lesson with us. At lunch and break times, we would be taken back to the library.

At first, it was only the three of us that had permission to be there. No friends allowed. But they weren't about to told that they couldn't join us. A mixture of nagging, talking to teachers, and phone calls from our parents to object to the fact that we were being isolated from our friends meant that we ended up with our own area of the library to socialise and feel safe.

When our friends were in there with us, we almost felt normal. My friend Laura was one of them, and she's still one of my best friends. I can only ever picture her smiling. Always making jokes, wearing brightly coloured shoes even though she wasn't supposed to, and talking about cute boys and bands. I thought she was one of the funniest, easiest people to speak to in the world. To me, she was so cool. And she didn't treat us like dirt. She laughed along with us, gave us nicknames and made us feel like people.

Laura would show up at the door of the library, we'd let her in, and she'd sneak us different sweets every few days. We would feast on Jaffa Cakes like stealthy ninjas. Sarah wasn't a girl of many words, but she would cheer us up drawing cartoons and giving sarcastic one-liners about the idiots we had to go to school with. She's still a good friend of ours today.

When the day was over, we had to go back to the library, wait until an hour after everyone had gone home, and only then would we be taken home by a teacher, or picked up by our heartbroken and guilt-ridden mother.

Enter again the charming Head of Year. He was unhappy with the fact that we were using the library so much, and especially unhappy that we were allowed to have company. He tried to change the arrangement, but a few phone calls from my parents soon changed that decision.

Stephanie was completely losing it by this point. One day, we had been sitting in the library for a while when we realised Steph wasn't sitting beside us. We found her sitting in between the shelves of books, as far back into the aisle as she could go, with her sandwiches in her hand. If she saw that Toni or I needed to go to the toilet, she would beg us to stay and wait until lesson time so that a teacher could come with us.

Every Friday afternoon, we would have a class which was next door to the form room of the boy who had caused this whole mess.

It was the black spot on my whole week's timetable. The countdown to the end of the lunch break was horrible. I would start to sweat and hear the blood pumping in my ears. Toni and I tried every week without fail to keep Stephanie distracted, but it didn't work.

Once, when we arrived at school and the caretaker hadn't opened the door, she had her first panic attack. She was sobbing and shouting and wouldn't stay still, running to try to find the nearest open door.

'What are we going to do? What are we going to do? What are we going to do?' she asked over and over again. 'They're going to get us.'

Toni took the role of the 'oldest'. She 'led' me and Steph at school, even though she was just as scared as us. She told me that the first day back at school after the attack, the sound of the school bell made her blood run cold. She made our decisions more often than not. We relied on her to sort everything out. I can't imagine now what that must have been like. It took me a lot of years to look back and recognise that for what it was.

We didn't have a life outside of school. We went home, we got a bath or shower, and we stayed behind closed doors until the next morning came around. When I heard the other kids at school talking about going out, or asking each other what time they were going to meet up that evening, I found it completely bizarre. We had tried a couple of times on the weekend to walk to our dad's house together, as he only lived a couple of streets away. The trouble was that a lot of those kids also lived on our estate. A group of them saw us, drove by repeatedly on their bikes and pelted us with stones as hard as they possibly could. We didn't leave the flat again all weekend. The anxiety and fear that we suffered at school had finally spread to our home life too.

We comfort ate – a lot. Steph hated buses, and any groups of more than two people. And I developed a fear that I didn't tell anybody about until I was in my early twenties – I was convinced that every time a car passed by, I would be shot. I would see a car in the distance, and the closer the car got to me, the tighter my muscles would tense up. I would close my eyes as the car approached me, and wait for the shot. I would feel surprised and relieved every time that it passed by without incident. And I went through the same ritual every time, dozens of times a week.

Our big sisters were noticing. One day, we had all gathered to see Nikki's new house that she had just moved into with her boyfriend and their kids. (Stephanie was refusing to leave the house at this point and was back at home by herself.) Nikki was literally halfway through explaining how she was going to decorate the living room when she stopped mid-sentence, looked at me and said, 'Oh Terri, I promise you it's going to be okay.' Natalie put her arms around me. I looked at them in surprise; I hadn't said anything. They told me that they could just see it in my face.

There was nothing else to do for the rest of our school life, except do our work and ride it out. We continued to be called fat, ugly, freaks, and, most annoyingly, twins. If these idiots were going to insult me, they could at least take the time to count to three. I hated every inch of my face and body by the time we left school. I was convinced that I had a stoop, flat hair, and a comically large nose. I was convinced that I was disgustingly fat.

I KNEW that I was going to fail all my exams, never find a boyfriend, and never fit in (happily, none of those things happened).

There were, surprisingly, some great things to come out of high school. We came away with some strong friendships, some of which survive to this day. But graduation couldn't come soon enough. When the headmistress said that she hoped one day that we would return to the school after graduation to give inspirational talks, the three of us laughed.

I knew I would never go back to that place unless I had to. But I couldn't stop myself ... and I found myself back there in anxiety dreams, going round and round the corridors, unable to find my way.

CHAPTER 5

IT'S THE END OF THE WORLD
AS WE KNOW IT - AND I FEEL FINE

When you get to 14 in Britain, you have to choose what subjects you study for the next two years, and it means dropping some other subjects. I enjoyed studying History and Geography, not least because I thought my teachers were fantastic. I admired intelligent people who had a strict approach to the idiots that would try to disrupt a class. And they did. But because I chose two humanities subjects, I had to drop French. When she heard, my French teacher came to speak to me personally: *why on earth was I dropping French? What a waste! I was really good at it!*

I remember being surprised. Was I that good? I knew I was doing well because I was doing relatively well across the board, but it was news to me that I was better at it than anyone else. She asked me to sit some mock exams to prove that she was right, and I scored an A* in all three.

Why hadn't I noticed my ability before? I was glowing with pride.

My French teacher helped me structure my options in a way that meant I could study History, Geography *and* French. Until then, I didn't really have any idea what I wanted to study after school, or what kind of career path I was going to take. But at least now I knew that I had some talent. So, what was there to lose?

I decided to see where it would take me if I applied myself outside of school too. I took a dictionary home. For the next few weeks, whenever I had an opportunity, I would look up random words. I would write long (and, in hindsight, cutely simple) passages in my diary in French. I bought an exam revision book and filled out all the exercises for fun. I translated conversations in my head.

My sisters and I, alongside our friends, all passed our GCSEs with excellent grades. Of course we did; we were clever. But we were also ridiculously uptight, worried, anxious, and panicky about exams, so we all revised like crazy. I remember many nights camping out together on our beds, dividing all our subjects three ways (because of course we all chose the same subjects). We made revision notes and flashcards, and took turns to rotate our notes and revise the other subjects.

I remember our physics teacher joking that we'd have to wear tinfoil hats during the exam so that we couldn't read each other's minds and cheat. If only.

We spent the time quizzing each other and bickering, panicking and reassuring each other. In amongst the pep talks, we would tell each other how worried we were about the undeniable fact that we were going to fail that subject, but how the others were going to get full marks.

I got an A* in French, and A–Cs in everything else. My sisters both did slightly better than me. (Why? Why was I less intelligent than them, dammit?) We looked at our college options, and – after briefly flirting with the idea of splitting up to go to separate places – all ended up choosing a local sixth form college.

Leaving high school was terrifying but liberating too. We attended the prom. I enjoyed the night with my friends, but felt sick watching all my classmates get dressed up and band together in huge swarms.

It was my first time in a social setting with them all, and I was really on edge. But, like everything else, it passed. And that was that ... the most challenging, heart-breaking, and terrifying five years of my young life were over just like that. It seemed anticlimactic.

That summer we turned 16, and I spent the holiday on French forums, chatting and exchanging language skills with French adolescents who wanted to learn English. I got even better at it. I found a pen pal, a boy called Quentin who lived in Caen. Up until then, I had learned French from books, teachers, and dictionaries. But this was a real-life person who would send me emails, pages, and pages long, about how life worked in France. When I replied, he didn't just understand, he was genuinely interested! I was speaking another language, legitimately! It was a wonderful feeling.

We looked forward to college but, of course, we were terrified too. It was one of our default settings by that point. The bullying wasn't over yet though. Some of them still lived in our neighbourhood, or knew people who did. We developed a system for catching buses; we would board, pay, and do a quick sweep of the seats to see if any of them were on board. We would rush to sit down before anyone could see us. And we'd choose the most strategic seats to avoid taunting, or the risk of being hit by any projectile pieces of food or whatever they had to throw at us.

The constant fear of waiting to be attacked or ridiculed was exhausting. My whole body would tense up and I would hold my breath. I'd feel a pain in my chest that was white-hot and freezing cold at the same time. I would sweat, and my eyes would fixate on one spot because I couldn't make myself look at the space around me and see who was there or what was happening. If I wanted to cry, my eyes would burn and my throat would constrict. I had lived with these feelings on and off for years; it never eased or got any more bearable.

I was extremely body conscious by now. It was a blazing hot summer, and I was covering up as much as possible. Walking into a supermarket one day with my mother, I refused to take off my thick black cardigan even though I felt like I was cooking alive. She told me not to be so silly and take it off. I could *not* do that. I was doing a public service. These were all innocent people – they hadn't come out on a Saturday to do a nice bit of shopping, only to see a half-dressed hippo sweeping its way through the aisles.

It was too warm to wear my long hair down, so I would tie it up into a ponytail, but not so high that I would violate bystanders' eyes with the sight of my Grandad turkey neck! Any time I saw a reflective surface that was so colossally big that it could show my entire reflection, I cringed away from the sight of my ginormous arse that stuck out so far it would enter a room a few minutes after I did. I cannot tell you how difficult it is to feel so conspicuous but want to hide away as much as possible. I felt like we stuck out like the three sore thumbs of a giant.

We were all still suffering the after-effects of years of bullying. Stephanie's fear of people and groups didn't simmer down. We were young; Toni and I were not as supportive as we could have been. We just didn't appreciate what was happening to her. There were times when we'd be walking down a street, and Steph would grab us and try to move us as close to the wall as possible. But we'd shrug her off. If she thought she saw anyone our age looking at us or talking about us, she started to repeat 'Oh no, oh no, oh no, oh no, oh no ...' We told her she was being an idiot, a maniac, or paranoid, until she would cry – and then we'd soften and try to comfort her. She would still beg us not to go anywhere if we didn't need to.

Day one of college came. I had been on a diet over the summer due to my ridiculously bad body issues, and I had lost some weight. Somebody snapped a phot of me a few days before the term started, and I was really surprised ... I actually looked quite slim.

Obviously, it was some lighting-angle-magic-camera kind of sorcery. But still, I looked a lot less like a humpback whale than I had a couple of months ago. So, I allowed myself to wear a white vest top and a knee length toffee-coloured skirt. I had newly highlighted my hair blonde.

Entering the building, I regretted the outfit immediately. The corridors were full of people. They were going to think I was *disgusting* and taunt me for it. The memory is still so vivid: I walked into a corridor that was glass-lined along one side, with a huge computer room. The people inside could see you passing as it you were in some sort of aquarium. I put myself as close to the wall as I possibly could, and diverted my line of sight to about a foot over everyone's heads.

But a few seconds in, I could sense that no one was staring at me. No one was making a beeline for me. No one was shouting insults at me. No one was throwing anything at me.

I was genuinely surprised. I could walk around like the rest of them, like I had the right to be here. The other kids weren't surprised that I was there, they weren't affronted by the fact that I was trying to act like a normal person. They didn't try to claim the space I was walking in. They didn't feel the need to remind me that I was fat and disgusting. No one called me a freak, or a nerd, or weird. And best of all, nobody wanted to physically hurt me.

For the next three years I can only remember happiness. I was studying the subjects I had really liked in school: French, History, English, and Psychology. My teachers were fun, the classes were interesting.

In high school, my friendships had been different. If there was a person willing to be nice to me who I found even slightly cool, it would almost not matter about the dynamics of the friendship. They could probably take more from the relationship than they gave, but I would let them because I was 'lucky' enough to even be counted as a friend. It wasn't healthy, and it was probably unbalanced. I think there was a small degree of hero worship too. But my low self-esteem had made that happen quite often.

In college, my friendships took on a different nature. Several of the people that stuck by us in those crappy library days came to the same college, and we remained friends. Over the space of the next two years, we kept our group together and added even more friends.

Laura, who lived a street away from me, became my best friend. She took Psychology too and between classes we spent all our time together. She made me laugh. We had the same sense of humour, and she was easy to be around. She was also different from me in a lot of ways – we didn't have the same dress sense, hobbies, taste in music, or even the same friends. But she shared everything with me. She introduced me to people she had met. She gave me her iPod on the bus ride to college, and I learned to like some of the bands she listened to. While I never picked it up, she started her driving lessons, and when she passed her test she ran and found me on the college bus, threw her certificate at me, and screamed, 'I passed!' I didn't feel a bitter jealousy; I was just genuinely happy she got what she wanted. She got a girly car, put sparkly pink stickers on it, and drove us to college every day. The small things made her happy.

Laura was a little beam of sunshine, and the laughter and enthusiasm made it difficult not to be cheerful around her. She gave me nicknames and tried to speak French with me because she knew I loved it. She asked me about my classes, my pen pal, my hobbies – and she asked because she was interested.

I remember being fascinated by Laura. She didn't flip out with nerves about exams or her driving lesson. I would ask everyone else if they were nervous before their exams – and when they said yes, I was delighted. I wasn't a freak then. It was normal for people to feel nervous. But I was still so envious of those who didn't.

While we studied at the same college, Toni, Steph, and I were starting to find more and more independence, and more differences between ourselves. Yes, we still bickered. Unbearably so. We were still in each other's pockets at home, on the commute to college, and even in our social group. But we had chosen to take some separate subjects which showed that, unlike high school, where we might have looked to be exactly the same from the outside, we were now finding our own passions.

Toni had discovered science, and chose to study biology and chemistry. Despite having done well in all my subjects, I achieved my lowest grades in science. I found it mind-boggling that not only did she choose to continue studying it, but that she was smart enough to do so. It solidified my opinion of Toni as so much smarter than me. I was in awe of it. And yes, I was jealous of it.

Steph had taken our mutual love of books and decided to go further with it, studying English language, literature, and philosophy. She became great with words, and began to read even more than ever. Very early on, she knew that she was going to work with words and books in some form or another. And to me, she fit into that role like a jigsaw piece. It just made sense. She was fantastic at helping me study grammar, to the point where I could understand my own native language in a way that made learning a foreign one even easier.

I signed up for extra French lessons and the favourite day in my whole week was Tuesday, when I would have four straight hours of French. The teacher was one of the best I had ever had. The lessons were excellent – we were allowed to gossip amongst ourselves as long as we did so in French. It was a small class, but these were *my* people. I made friends with a boy called Sam. Mrs Cogan (my high school teacher) may have been the reason that I had made it this far in my French-speaking career, but I would say that Sam was the one who influenced me into keeping it going into adulthood.

Sam would spend break times showing me comedy videos in French, and I would be amazed and ecstatic that I could understand them. For practise, we would sit and speak in French socially.

Once our French teacher told us that a local high school was looking for French-speaking students to help out at a French-themed day. The children would have fake passports, board 'flights', and land in 'France', where they would then speak French, sing French songs, dress like French people, see the French tourist sights, and eat French food.

By lunchtime, Sam and I had eaten so much garlic French cheese that we were paranoid about having terrible breath. We cracked so many jokes about our garlic breath that we were in fits of laughter. A man came and sat next to us and, in all of our cockiness, we began to talk in French about beautiful he was, and how disappointed we were that we both had cheese breath. He was so cute. Why hadn't we held off on eating all that Roulé? What if he wanted to talk to one of us?

A couple of hours and a few sticks of desperately needed extra strong chewing gums later, Sam and I were in the staff room. The guy walked in, introduced himself, and shook our hands. Cue the knowing smirks. We got talking, and he explained that he was there because he knew one of the teachers, who'd invited him because he had lived and studied in France for several years. And of course, he was fluent in French! He got up to make a drink. Sam quickly wrote something down and slipped the note to me across the table.

'FUUUUUUUUUUUUUUUUUUUUUUUUCK.'

And that was how I learned not to assume that the people around me don't understand what I'm saying. I don't know about Sam, but I have been extra careful about it ever since!

In one of our classes, the conversation came around to studies after college. I hadn't made any decisions, or, I believe, allowed myself to give it much thought. I was happy here and thinking about having to leave wasn't the best thought in the world. Sam told me that he had chosen a degree at the University of Hull.

I asked him, 'Are you going to study French?'

'Not just French. I'm going to do a degree called Combined Languages. I'm going to pick up German too.'

I knew that alongside French, he also studied Spanish at college. A few people in my class actually studied more than one language, and I had long since been jealous that I'd never had the opportunity to learn more than one.

'You can pick up another language without doing it at school?'

I was stunned. In school, the teachers had had an uncanny talent of making you feel like you would either have to pass your exams and go to college, or leave school and have to face the apocalypse! They certainly hadn't told us there was a whole world of things you could do at degree level without having done them at school first.

'Of course you can!' he told me. 'You just need to have studied one language to A-Level standard. It's a four-year degree, and in your third year you get to travel and work or study abroad. You should do it. You can pick up more than one language, you know.'

No, Sam, I didn't know. But I did now. That night I went home and read about the course on the university website. It promised four years of language learning, and, not only that, I could be like the people I had envied for so long and learn to speak even more than one. And so, just like that, the next few years of my life suddenly had a direction.

The first year of university was incredibly exciting. I had chosen to study French, Spanish, and Italian. The campus was huge compared to the tiny little college I'd come from, and the atmosphere was fantastic. It was a new start – exciting but safe. I was going to be here for the next four years studying something I loved, and making new friends – something I finally knew I was good at. There were no threats. I felt free.

The second year of university quickly swung around, and with it, lots of brand-new experiences. I had decided to move into a student house with some friends that I had made in the first year – it was my first time living away from home. We chose a house a few yards away from the campus, a stone's throw from where my classes were held, and within view of the university bar and nightclub.

I had also fallen in love in the summer before the academic year started and we were soon spending all of our time together. I loved his family, especially his mother. I loved her genuinely and dearly, and she treated me like a daughter. His father had a great sense of humour and I loved spending time with them all.

He was my first boyfriend and I fell for him in that kind of dramatic, honeymoon kind of first love. He got along with my university friends like a house on fire, and we had a fun year of parties, day trips and film nights that I'll never forget. When I told him that I was going abroad for my third academic year, we agreed to stay together and try a long-distance relationship for the 13 months that I would be away.

CHAPTER 6

EVERYBODY HURTS

Mental illness can present itself differently in each person. Out of curiosity, I once asked Toni what anxiety meant for her. It meant worrying, obviously, but how had it affected her life? She was brutally honest about it:

Anxiety for me is a constant background level of dread or doom, trying not to think about something that is always in the back of your mind and never goes away. When I open a letter or an email that's about something that stresses me, it feels like someone has just grabbed my throat or squeezed my heart. It gives you tension headaches that feel like a gritty soreness behind the eyes. It makes you feel like there is a big hurdle in front of you and you can't think or contemplate anything beyond a certain time, event, or deadline. It becomes impossible to enjoy anything because you can't focus on anything properly. It makes you look at other people and seriously envy or resent them for having the freedom of going to eat a meal or watch a movie without any pressure on them. It paralyses you from taking any action because you feel like the only thing worse than the anticipation of a scary situation is the outcome itself, even though this hardly ever turns out to be true. Your mind cannot fathom things ending well.

It makes you feel useless and stupid and talentless. You feel incapable. You naturally become a pessimist because you feel like there will always be something to dread in life. You even start to picture your whole life worrying because you know there will be future presentations, job interviews, and exams coming up for the rest of your life.

If you go to sleep thinking about whatever you're worried about, you wake up with your heart racing in your throat. You have an inner monologue of 'You are useless and you are wasting your life putting everything off.'

Time becomes a big source of discomfort, because you are acutely aware of time you are spending doing things that aren't meaningful. You do it in order to avoid what is stressing you out the most – usually an important project like a job search or a big change in your life.

Sometimes, I'll read an article or a blog about something that I experience in my own life. If it's in a book, I fold down the page to go back to it later, because it speaks to me. I once read a book called *The Amazing Adventures of Dietgirl* by Shauna Reid, where an Australian lady spoke about the battle against her own willpower to fight obesity. That book is, ironically, now twice the size because it's bulked out from folded pages. When I see things online, I 'bookmark' the page to come back to later. It amazes me to read about other people who experience feelings the same way as me.

So, it's still a mystery to me how I can be surprised that my own sister has had the same struggles as me. Reading this back, it's still fascinating how exact her description of it is. I've had all these symptoms and more, and this is probably just the tip of the iceberg for her too.

When I asked Steph, though, her experience was different from mine, but no less painful:

Feeling anxious is like having a little itch that you can't scratch. It's like your chest and face are on fire, like something has massively upset you but you can't think what, which makes you feel like you can't begin to fix it. Anxiety has given me something called trichotillomania. It's an anxiety induced condition that makes me want to pull my eyebrows out (for *others it can be hair from the head or face). The NHS characterises it as 'a psychological condition where the person is unable to stop themselves carrying out a particular action'. It makes me feel guilty and embarrassed and unattractive, and because it's on such a visible part of my body, I am constantly worrying about people noticing. It is a huge knock to my self-esteem.*

Anxiety makes my head feel cloudy, and when I'm at my worst, I can't focus on anything. It feels like there's an invisible wall in front of me that I can't get past. I can't accomplish anything until I figure out how to climb over it.

Anxiety can make me cut myself off from my friends and family because I don't want them to know that I don't always function well and that I can sometimes let things in my life go to shit before sorting them out again. If I was spinning plates, and one of the plates fell, I'd let them all drop to the floor before trying to get any of them spinning again.

Sometimes it has me clawing or scratching at my arms and legs without realising I've even done it. It makes me pretend to the outside world that I'm doing everything fine when I feel like I'm doing everything wrong.

These are just summaries of the things my sisters have had to learn to overcome. Here are my experiences in a little more detail. There are a lot of overlaps. Maybe there will be for you too. Maybe you'll even get to fold some pages along the way …

CHAPTER 7

CAN'T GET THERE FROM HERE

I'd had a brief break from anxiety in social situations at college and in the first two years of university. But I was still experiencing uncontrollable nerves and freak-outs when it came to exams.

For now, I was still in the protective bubble of my academic years: I knew exactly where I was going to be at the end of a summer break, where to register, which books to buy, which classes to show up to, and which exams I would be sitting. The outside world wasn't an issue because I had a set structure and set rules to live by. As long as I did my revision and passed my exams, I was good, so I knew that was where my anxiety was rooted.

I was already dreading the last year when I would take the exams that would determine how I would spend the next few years of my life. Would I get the jobs I wanted or look back on failed exams, saying 'Oh, well, at least I had some fun,' while looking at old photos and reminiscing about the time I fell asleep hugging a takeaway?

The Big Wide World was looming. There were all of these new opportunities to be a complete failure. Before, the biggest risk was failing a few exams or disappointing a few teachers. Now I could see myself ending up in a dead-end job, not living up to the expectations that I convinced myself my parents must have had for me.

But, for a little longer, I was still safe. I was still in the cocoon. Naïvely, I thought I had left my big problems behind in high school and they were never going to find me again.

I did not emerge from that safe cocoon as a butterfly. The next two years I was more like a haggard moth.

It was my year abroad, a time to immerse myself in the foreign languages that I was studying for my degree. And because I was learning three languages, I had to split the year between all three countries. Even for the most well-adjusted of students, it was a scary thing, but exciting too.

It wasn't scary for me ... It was terrifying. I spent the whole summer counting down the days to my departure date, but not for the right reasons.

What if I got kidnapped? What about my boyfriend? I was in love and he looked after me all the time. How could I leave him? Would we still be together at the end of it? What if I got kidnapped? Who the hell was going to help me? Would my friends get bored and forget about me while I was out there? What if I got there and realised that my language skills were a pile of crap? What if I ran out of money? What if I got kidnapped miles away from home? What if I didn't make any friends? *What if I got kidnapped?*

In the run-up to the year abroad we were having monthly meetings with a department called the international office. We would talk about the logistics of travelling, our job choices, our university applications, the financial side of things, etc. However, there was also the personal and emotional side of things to consider, and we were given fair warning about how difficult it would be to move to a foreign country. (And by fair warning, I mean that there was a letter containing a two-line comment that said: *In the first two weeks of your stay in your host country, you will want to come home. You must stick it out – this will be from the culture shock and it will subside once you have got your bearings.)*

They weren't wrong. Country one: Italy. I was worried about the language barrier (I had only done two years of Italian and Spanish, and it was expected that I should now be at the same level as my classmates who had been studying these languages for years). It was a situation rife with opportunities for self-comparison and putting myself down! I didn't even have anywhere to live lined up when I boarded the plane. The idea was that we would land and then sort out the accommodation.

I boarded the flight with a girl called Kim. I didn't know her that well, but liked her well enough. We hadn't spent a lot of time together socially, but banded together to look after each other while we travelled. I even managed to worry about whether we'd talk easily enough because I knew we would be clinging to each other like barnacles in the first few weeks. I needn't have worried – Kim was even chattier than I was and had a way of putting a funny edge on even the most ridiculous situations that we got ourselves into. She reminded me of one of those people that, had we been in a sitcom, the camera would have cut to her for a reaction every time something weird, silly, awkward, or confusing happened. She kept me laughing in some of the scariest times.

We landed in the small city of Perugia. The university was classed as a university of foreigners, and named as such: Università per Stranieri. To me, the citizens of Perugia did NOT seem happy to be a city for foreign students. To me, it felt like the village from the film *Hot Fuzz* – that Simon Pegg movie in which a police officer moves from the Met force in London to a sleepy little village where the residents resent newcomers and outsiders. I knew something didn't feel right, but I just didn't know what. For me, that feeling was stronger than it was for the other girls from my classes. I certainly seemed to be a lot more homesick than they were, or, at least, I wasn't coping with it as well as they were.

Most people I knew from my courses had at least left their hometowns to come to Hull uni – but I had never left the safety of my birthplace. I hadn't had to make friends completely from scratch, without anyone with me, in years. Even when I'd had to do it as a kid, I was never completely alone because of Toni and Stephanie. This was my first time living anywhere other than Hull.

As I said, we didn't have a clue what we were supposed to be doing. All we knew is that we had to go to a little office for foreigners, which was like the equivalent of our international office.

In our first contact with the Italian people, we encountered the most delightful specimen of a human being. He looked like the little old guy from the Disney film *Up*, but much less cheerful. He was screaming as we walked in. The door was propped open and a couple of girls went in, one after the other, and then came out looking really tearful.

At that point, Kim looked at me with horror in her eyes. Who was this tiny Disney man, and why did he want us dead? He came out, and we knew our doom had arrived.

We stood up, he looked at us and screamed 'Passaporte!'

We followed him into his office and I can honestly say that I could not understand a word that he was shrieking in our direction. He seemed to alternate between being angry with us for even daring to exist, and running an open monologue where he seemed to be asking himself questions and answering them within the same breath. He hardly stopped to draw breath, only intermittently looking over at us for an answer. Then we just looked back at him in stunned amazement, while crickets chirped and tumbleweed rolled across the room, as we waited for his fury to unfurl at not being understood.

We did not have a clue what was going on, or what mistakes we had made in our half-hour of being residents in his city, to merit him being so pissed off. Eventually I just told him in nervous Italian that we had no idea where we needed to go, and all we had were the documents in front of us.

He tutted in disgust and scribbled down a few letters on a piece of paper: 'v. del fav.' We were so relieved the meeting was over that we just left the office. We came out of the building into a square, sat down on some nearby benches, and tried to make sense of what he had written down.

We couldn't. We ended up dragging two suitcases each, up cobbled hills back to the office to find out. It was closed. We went back into the square into a local newsagent. This was 2010, the days of yore, where we did not have 4G, and we had to find ye olde streets on ye olde ancient map.

On ye olde map, we found a local youth hostel where we decided to stay for the night. It took us another couple of hours; at one point, we were led down what I thought was an alleyway by a stranger who had grabbed one of our suitcases in order to 'help' us find the hostel. The buildings were so close to each other at the top that they were almost touching, and hardly any light was coming through.

Kim signalled to me that she was pretty sure we were going to die. I grabbed the suitcase back and thanked the man for his kind help, but that we'd had a sudden stroke of genius halfway through the alley and knew exactly where we needed to go. An hour later we found the stranger who had tried to help us sitting outside a little café a few yards away from the hostel that he had clearly been trying to lead us to to begin with.

We stayed the night in the hostel and dreaded going back to our lovely friend in the international office. The next day, we got our courage up and found Mr. Disney, who shouted 'Via del Favarone!' at us until a lady explained that that was the street name where our dormitory was.

Kim kept up an angry 'Oh well, of course that's what v. del fav means, how can we not have known that?' Then we were driven around the hilly city in a tiny little Fiat Cinquecento by a strange man who wasn't much happier than Mr. Disney.

Because of this traumatic reception, we were nervous about dealing with the international office again. There was a lot of paperwork to get done, including a form that the office had to sign to attest that we had shown up and checked in, and therefore we were eligible for our grants and tuition money.

We went back with two girls from our university and stood outside, trying to talk each other into going in and asking the staff to sign our paperwork. We were really nervous because we thought that if the staff asked us any technical questions, we wouldn't have a clue how to answer them in passable Italian. In my head, I knew that I was barely saying anything and acting quite stoic, determined just to laugh along when needed, and not let on to the girls that I was nervous.

It was normal to be nervous – of course it was, and I didn't judge them for being open about it. I was actually really jealous at how comfortable they were telling each other how they were feeling, and how easily they could laugh it all off. I wasn't comfortable enough to do the same.

We bottled it that first time, but the other girls had managed to get their forms signed. Out of fear, I just plain and simply didn't go and get it done. Over the next few weeks I kept putting it off, and the situation just got worse and worse. I got to the point where I was even too scared to ask Kim if she'd had hers signed in case she asked why I hadn't got mine done.

This was my first experience of one of the worst anxiety symptoms I have struggled with: avoidance coping.

Avoidance coping can come in two forms: active avoidance, or passive avoidance. When actively avoiding something, you take measures to prevent a certain fear or situation from coming to pass. We see this a lot in people suffering from OCD, who believe that they must wash excessively to avoid exposure to germs, for example.

I am the master of passive avoidance. I just don't act upon a situation that is threatening me – I attempt to completely ignore it, hide it, or deny its very existence because I can't deal with the fear. Of course, it doesn't work. My 'comfort zone' is the least comfortable place in the world. I don't face the situation at hand in order to avoid the bad feelings it would cause in me. But the constant worrying about it is almost worse.

I was attempting complete denial. But the worry was like a black tornado whirling around silently inside me where nobody could see it. It was quite literally painful. My heart slammed in my chest and I was getting intense headaches from the stress. I got to the point where I would be thinking about the fear – in this instance the paperwork and the belief that I was going to lose my grants and tuition – several times a day. I was carrying around a feeling of pure dread.

If I thought about it before I went to sleep, which was most of the time, I would dream about it. Sometimes I would jolt awake, terror gripping my chest, and the subject would jump into my head. It was like waking up and remembering a nightmare.

I knew that at any point I could – and should – go and sort it out. Every day that I left it was potentially making the situation worse. I knew that. But the paralysing fear meant that even though the situation was getting more and more out of hand, I could not bring myself to action it and face the reality of what a failure I had been.

I was always waiting for night to fall. Because you know that when you are lying in bed on a dark night, and the curtains are closed and the door is locked, everybody else is asleep. And because everybody is asleep, nobody is expecting anything from you. Nobody is out there judging you. Nobody is sitting there and waiting for that form. That is when you can lie in bed, be your own hero in your own head, and tell yourself that you are going to be the best version of yourself that you have ever been. When the sun comes up, you are going to fix everything. You congratulate yourself because the solution that you have come up with is so genius and then you can go to sleep.

And then, the next morning hits, and the sun comes up. Everyone else is awake, and they could be thinking about you, and thinking about how you've let them down. And then reality hits and you realise what an idiot you've actually been. What seemed like a fantastic idea the night before suddenly makes no sense whatsoever.

Physically, I buried the form. It went into a paper envelope, inside a folder, inside some clothes, inside a suitcase and under the bed. It was like a bad secret that was banished to where I couldn't see it, and it couldn't hurt me. But, every time I would walk into the room, my eyes would immediately shoot over to the bed. My line of sight was always drawn to it.

I was waiting for the day that it would come to light, and somebody would tell me that I hadn't done it, that I was going to get kicked off my course. I would have to go home from my year abroad and it would be all my fault for not getting the paperwork done. I was convinced that it was going to happen, but I was still so scared of admitting what I had done wrong. I already knew that I was fat and ugly. If I was going to be seen as a failure as well, then what self-esteem was I going to have left?

I was too scared to open my emails. I wouldn't even log on in case someone was asking about it. This made things easier and harder. My imagination was telling me that people were emailing me and getting angry. I dreaded the call coming from my supervisor. I remember trying to sleep at night and thinking that, if I had to choose between getting a boat load of money or having the situation magically solved, I would choose for the situation to be solved. Every time.

Some nights I would dream that it had all been sorted out, and then, when I woke up, I would be crushed when I realised it hadn't.

The anxiety didn't stop … On the day we were supposed to sit our exams, we went into the class and saw another 120 students! We realised that they had to give their exams in front of the other students, and do them verbally. At that time, the only way we could have sat an Italian exam would have been a written exam that we could correct as we went along. We didn't have that option.

I was facing the prospect of sitting at front of the room, with the spotlight on me and my subpar language skills, and talking about art. In Italian! I struggle to talk about art in English – I had nothing.

Emma burst into hysterical and infectious giggles. Kim, with her knack of saying what everyone was thinking, declared:

'There's no way we can do this. What do they want from us?'

We went to a bar. Kim called the international office back home and explained our predicament. If we couldn't do it, were we going to fail our degrees? The office said they would work with us to find another way for us to be assessed.

While they were on the phone, they casually mentioned the form. 'You might not have a copy of it, I'll email you over a new copy and you can get it signed.'

And that was it. In the space of a few seconds this person – who I didn't even know said two sentences that immediately ended months of torment. Hannah was joking and saying 'It's 11am! Too early for a cocktail?'

It wasn't. I sat in the bar, staring at my glass, my face frozen in a stunned smile. My face and chest felt cold and yet I could feel myself blushing. My hands were shaking; my body just did not know how to react. I think it must have been relief.

Does this all sound ridiculous to you? Have you read this and thought, if only just for a second, 'This girl's going a bit overboard,' or 'That's a bit of an overreaction,' or even 'How childish'? Then this is something you must understand: this is what anxiety does. It makes you overreact.

Your problems can be molehills, but instead of being able to walk over them in one stride, anxiety turns you into this tiny person who can only see mountains. You don't have the mental facilities to see the problem for what it actually is, and the gravity of it can take over your whole world. (And the more people label you as childish, paranoid, or negative, the more you feel like you can't tell people what's going on.)

I never assume I know what's going on inside a person's head. I try to make my judgements on a person's intentions, not on one single action. People are rarely 'just being' a certain way for the hell of it. Labels are dangerous. We should all try to consider the reasons why someone may be acting strangely, immaturely, or whatever generalised conclusion we might otherwise come up with.

Nobody can be summed up in one negative word. Because when you hear it from someone else, it stays with you. Sometimes, it backs up some negative feelings that you already have about yourself. Long after they've forgotten ever saying it, you will still be playing it in your head.

I know now that this incident wasn't just about a form. My anxiety was getting worse, and this was just one of the ways that it was coming out. This kind of avoidance has happened to me more than once since. I have ignored situations that have been distressing me for weeks on end, every night going to sleep telling myself that the next day would be the one that I would face it, action it, solve it. When you're anxious, you can be sitting completely still, with nowhere to go and nowhere to be, but your whole body is jittery while your mind tells you there is something you should be doing, somewhere you should be going, someone you need to speak to, a problem you need to solve.

When you try to relax, you feel like it's not safe to. Hundreds of times I sat down to knit or read – anything to help me relax – but I would be feeling guilty while doing it because I didn't feel I had earned the right to be relaxing when there were so many broken areas of my life I needed to fix.

By the time I got back to Hull, I had changed in a lot of ways. There were the good changes …

I had learned to do the sorts of things that I would never in a million years have had the guts to do if I hadn't been obliged to go out there and do them. For example, I was a lot more confident in meeting and speaking with new people. I could travel independently (I still speak of the year I took 16 flights), and my languages had improved. My friends and my parents had come to visit me in Paris, and some of them had said that the way I held myself around my colleagues and moved myself around the big city with ease was inspiring to see. These were the good things.

But when I got back and moved into a house with three of my closest friends, they started seeing the negative differences. And they were qualified to pick up on it – we had been really close before I went away and they were there waiting for me when I came back. I was less jokey, less cheerful, less chatty – all of the characteristics that had attracted friends, and especially my boyfriend, to me to begin with.

Cheerful, shiny, happy Terri – as I knew – her was gone. I had a heavier aura about me. I was more irritable and more prone to starting arguments.

I couldn't explain it to anyone. I hadn't noticed it too much myself. For me, the change had been much more gradual. For those around me, a pleasant person had boarded the plane and a bit of grouch had come back in her place.

Don't get me wrong, I still had a lot of good times while I was there, but I had gone through some really tough emotions on my year abroad that I hadn't experienced to that degree before. You're supposed to come back and rave about how excellent every moment of it was. It's not adventurous, or exciting, or exotic to say that you were homesick all the time, and you couldn't wait to get back to all the comfortable things in your life. (The crap bacon alone was enough to make me want to pack up and come home.)

The fact is that I wasn't as happy in my final year of university as I had been in my first two. And with the end of my time at uni looming, things were starting to feel threatening. Life and all of its potential bitch-slaps were looking all too real.

When my studies picked back up, I remember thinking that I simply couldn't cope with the new workload. It felt like an avalanche had hit and all you could see of me from underneath was the top of my flaming red hair. The intensity of the work had stepped up massively, and everyone was feeling the strain – I don't really think there had been a steady transition between the workload that we had experienced in the previous years and what we were dealing with now.

At that point, it didn't seem realistic to think that I could continue with three foreign languages and pass my degree with a decent grade. At first, I dealt with it all wrongly. Avoidance came dancing in. I skipped a few classes. I was giving myself 'valid excuses' – I was trying to convince myself that I had good reasons for not going. For example, if I skipped a Spanish lesson I could tell myself that I had woken up too late, when in reality, if I had rushed myself along a little bit more, I know I could have made it. Alternatively, I would tell myself that a piece of work for another class was much more urgent and my time would be better spent doing that instead.

After a while, I started to realise that if I was going to continue like this then my degree was going to suffer significantly. I had done too much and worked too hard to let this turn into another one of those things I just ignored.

I'm still proud to this day that I came to this realisation. I didn't let avoidance win out. I went straight to my supervisor and asked if there was any chance of restructuring my degree to do the two languages. Could I pick up some history or cultural modules for one of the other languages instead?

I had decided on keeping French and Italian. I know in hindsight that this probably wasn't the best move – the more widely used language of the three is Spanish. I have even kept it going in my post-university career and social life, unlike Italian.

But even this was a decision grounded in low self-belief. With Italian, I felt that I was on the same level ability-wise with my classmates. We had all entered uni as complete beginners, and I felt less intimidated as a result. With Spanish, I felt so inferior to everybody else when I was in a classroom with them. It was a horrible feeling that became a loud background noise that interfered with my learning.

I therefore asked to keep Italian, with the benefit being that the Head of Combined Language herself was an Italian lady who I believe was happy that I wanted to continue with her lessons. She was a brilliant woman who managed to restructure my degree title and my modules so that I could continue my degree for the final year, one language down.

Yes, I was proud, but I was determined to be quietly proud about it. I didn't tell any of my classmates – I just stopped showing up. Until one day, I saw Sam from French class on the way to a Spanish history class. We were laughing along together when I had to stop at the door to my class. He walked forward a few paces, before turning around and saying:

'Aren't you coming to Spanish class?'

I took a deep breath and made the decision not to lie. I am ashamed of how many seconds it took me to make that decision, but I couldn't cope with telling him a bare-faced lie.

'Look, I haven't said anything because I'm quite embarrassed about it, but I dropped Spanish because at this level I just wasn't coping with doing three full languages at once.'

Rather than judging me, he told me that he thought that I had been brave. He thought a lot of people would probably wish they'd been brave enough to restructure their degrees, because it was taking its toll on other people too.

I don't know if he even remembers saying it to me, but I still remember it, five years later. It stayed with me because it's what I really needed to hear at the time.

By this stage, I had already skipped a few French classes. This had been sparked by a comment that the teacher made about an essay I had written. It was completely anonymous work and so I wasn't singled out, but still, something that I had written had been repeated and mocked in front of a classroom full of my friends and colleagues. I had been mortified and heartbroken at the time; the teacher was my favourite and I had looked up to him ever since I started the degree. I had struggled through the rest of the class with tears in my eyes. French was the only subject that I didn't constantly doubt myself over, and now I had suffered a huge blow to the fragile ego it gave me.

I had skipped so many of those classes that I'd developed a fear of walking through the modern foreign languages corridor where all the teachers were based. I remember approaching the corridor and keeping my eyeline fixed on the other end – I would walk through it as quickly as my tubby legs would carry me before the teachers could spot me.

If my friends were with me and they stopped to look at the notice board, I would make an excuse and go to the toilet. I was so nervous about running into one of the teachers whose classes I wasn't attending any more, and of course, inevitably, one day it happened. My teacher caught sight of me, and looked at me with huge concern on his face.

'Terri! Hello! I've been worried about you, where have you been?'

I understood his confusion. He didn't think it was like me to skip lessons. I had signed up for extra grammar classes for Christ's sake. I was 'one of those.'

I must have looked like a clown with the bright hair and the stupid smile that I plastered on my face. I don't remember what I said, except that it was a bunch of non-committal sentences that didn't mean anything. I wasn't about to give anything away. I felt hurt and angry with myself. This was a teacher and a class that I loved. But I had left it too long to feel like I could just walk in and pick it back up – I was so scared to have to try to explain that I wasn't a failure.

CHAPTER 8

BEACH BALL

I left university a year later than my sisters because of the year I spent abroad. By the time I graduated, Toni had been working in a hotel for a while, a job that she hated. The boss was a complete bully – berating her for the slightest things and humiliating her in front of guests by publicly pointing out what she had done wrong. She decided to leave the job for her own sanity.

Stephanie was working in a small CD and DVD shop on £7.50 an hour. I had been job searching for a couple of months and nothing had come up. Stephanie's boss suggested that we give in our CVs and do some part time work with them, and that was the start of a two-year stint of the three of us working together.

In all of the campaigns that aim to make society more aware of depression and anxiety, it's highlighted that these are invisible illnesses. A person can look physically healthy, but still be in real, desperate trouble in their minds, while those around them are completely oblivious to it. What happens behind closed doors sometimes doesn't come to public sight until it's too late, or until something extreme happens.

Sometimes though, it's not so invisible. When you're close enough to someone – because you live with them, you're in a relationship with them, or you're responsible for them – there will be signs.

There will be cries for help, and they can come out in a million different ways.

We're told to look out for the big, easily telegraphed signs: anorexic people who are painfully thin, alcoholics who are never without a drink in hand, depressed people who have put blades to their skin to let out some of the pain. Many signs aren't so extreme, but they are no less real, and they cause even more worries for the person suffering. I have seen people pull out their hair, bite their nails to the quick, and develop anxious ticks.

They're all physical ways of dealing with anxiety and depression. They can provide a distraction from emotional pain by replacing it with physical pain, e.g. self-harming. They can give you something that you feel you have control over when the rest of your life is spinning out of your control, e.g. an eating disorder. Some just give you that temporary rush of feel-good chemicals which, over time, push you to need more and more to get the same feeling, e.g. addictions.

For me, the physical manifestations came out in the form of binge eating. I don't mean offering out slices of pizza to my friends (while daring them to accept) and then eating the whole thing myself while laughing and declaring myself 'a fatty'.

Binge eating, in the truest, most extreme sense of the term, is not something that you do socially, or around people you love. No matter how much you share with them, it is very much a solo activity. I am yet to speak to anybody or read about anybody that has ever done it in company. It is something that you feel very embarrassed and ashamed about at the time.

My worst phase of binge eating when I lived with my dad. During my year abroad, my mother and sisters had moved from my childhood home to a smaller house up the road. When I'd finished my final year of uni, there wasn't a bedroom for me to take, but Dad had a spare room that I could use.

The anxiety was back. I'd had four years at university, but now I wasn't doing anything even close to what I thought I should be doing with my life. It's easy to spend years of your life telling yourself that when you leave education and get out into the Big Wide World you are going to conquer the job market, get the role of your dreams, and be successful. But the reality for some can be really daunting when the time finally comes to put those goals into action. Suddenly these things weren't for Future Terri to worry about any more, they were for me to sort out.

I had the spiel all planned out. When people I knew would see me in the shop, my defence was locked and loaded and ready to go: I was looking into teaching, I was putting applications out, I was keeping my options open, and spending all of my free time researching what to do next. I think at the time, I was hoping and praying that I was convincing people. In hindsight, I don't think I was fooling anybody. What I don't know is how much anyone was aware that it was because of crippling self-doubt and the white-hot fear of trying, not plain laziness and complacency.

I would like to tell the reader this: if there is something that you have been meaning to do for a long time, something that either you or the people around you think that you should be doing with your life, and you haven't, please don't automatically call yourself lazy. As Peter would say, this is the voice of The Judge – it's an unhelpful self-criticism that doesn't serve anything except to make you feel worse. I would ask others to always ask themselves, before calling anybody lazy, whether there is a possibility that fear is in play somewhere, acting as a barrier. It is highly likely that you aren't lazy at all – you are just scared of failing. If you don't try, you can't fail and you can't tell yourself you're useless for not being able to succeed. Of course, this horrible double-edged sword means that you end up calling criticising yourself for something else completely – you are a failure for not trying. Anxiety and low self-esteem will always find a way to make you self-hate.

So, I worked part time, yes, but I wasn't going home and spending all my time applying for jobs. Dad worked full-time, and so did my boyfriend. I was going home and, between seeing friends, I was secretly eating everything that came into my path.

I loved the people, I loved my bosses, but I didn't get any self-esteem from work. I had always been regarded as intelligent and accomplished. I had just finished a four-year degree – putting myself into thousands of pounds worth of debt – and now, I was flushing it all down the toilet. I didn't have the emotional health or clarity of mind to tell myself that I was just a matter of months out of university, and it was okay not to have anything figured out yet.

I was paranoid that people thought I had taken a job with my sisters because I couldn't be away from them. As much as I loved them, nothing could have been further from the truth – hadn't I just lived in three foreign countries without them? But whenever the three of us saw the familiar face of someone we used to know, or someone we'd lost touch with, one of us would stealthily sneak into the back room. (Okay, I admit it probably wasn't stealthy for me at the huge size I had reached.)

That much anxiety and fear and disappointment had to come out in some way. It's like a pressure valve – I think I would have exploded if I didn't have an outlet for the feelings.

What that essentially means is this: I was feeling down, and the stress was building. I wasn't getting fulfilment at work. I wasn't having the same level of happiness in my relationship with my partner anymore because we were arguing so much. I was an anxious, argumentative nightmare to live with. I didn't smile and laugh like I used to when we first met. And he couldn't begin to understand what was happening, or how to deal with it properly.

The quickest, most direct way for me to make myself feel better – to get that dopamine rush – was to eat massively. I didn't smoke, I didn't take drugs or anything like that, so my vice was food. Sometimes it was because of a trigger – an argument with my boyfriend, seeing an old university friend who was doing better than I was ... anything that made me upset. Sometimes, it was simply because the flat was empty and there was an opportunity to eat.

There was never any build up to it. It was always a snap decision. I didn't stop to consider the pros or cons, there wasn't any reasoning involved. I could have been sitting and watching the TV, or I could have just walked through the door.

Now, Dad wasn't an overeater, but he certainly never lived off what he liked to call 'rabbit food.' There was always lots of chocolate in the house for when the grandkids came over. But chocolate was not my poison. I loved savoury food: pastry, bread, crisps, you name it. I could eat it like it was the apocalypse. He always had thick doorstop bread, full fat milk, thick butter, sausage rolls, bacon, and multipacks of crisps. The fact that he could have them in the house and they'd still be there a week, two weeks, three weeks later was nothing short of sorcery to me! It didn't make sense. How could he eat something small for his evening meal, sit in his living room, and then not eat anything else for the rest of the night? It was all just sitting in the cupboards and the fridge in the next room, and he could just leave it there!

But it was like a trance would come over me – I would have a few moments of being completely shut off from my negative feelings. Or any feelings at all, in fact.

It was nothing to do with the quality of the food. Actually, junk food gave me a faster sugar high. I would start with a multipack of crisps, shoving in handfuls so quickly I barely even tasted them. I would toast my way through a few slices of bread, and eat three sausage rolls while I waited. A few slices in, I would lose patience with waiting for it to toast and end up buttering the bread and eating it that way. When I even lost patience with that, dry bread would follow.

Because there was always lots of food in the house, bingeing sessions were almost too easy to disguise. It felt like a crime scene clean-up afterwards. I would hide all of the evidence that it had ever happened. Sometimes, I would have to go to the local shop to replace a loaf of bread that I had managed to wolf my way through. If the bread had already been open when I had eaten it, I would get rid of a couple of slices, so I didn't have to explain to my dad how we were in possession of a magically self-replenishing loaf. Sometimes, that was a bonus – more to eat – and this time, I had to. But other times, I just had to throw it in the bin because I had made myself feel that sick.

Washing the kitchen, cleaning the bowls and throwing out the empty wrappers offered some sense of wiping away the sin, but the stabbing stomach cramps and waves of sickness couldn't be ignored. I felt as if I was the size of a bus. The high of eating lasted 20 minutes, the pure self-disgust lasted for hours, or days. And, what was the best way to feel better when you felt that low? I was pretty sure we still had some sausage rolls left ...

That October, we dressed in Halloween outfits in the shop. We had a witch, a princess, a wrestler, even Jack Skellington from *The Nightmare Before Christmas*, complete with stilts. I came downstairs with a white painted face, a red cape, fangs, and fake blood on my mouth. I thought that I had come as a vampire – but looking at the photos now, I looked more like a cannibal vampire that had eaten Dracula, his family, and all of his friends. I was the shape of a beach ball.

So, how do I feel now, after sharing the undignified, no-holds-barred truth with you all? The instinct is to feel embarrassed. I'm living in a world where telling people the number that appears on the bathroom scale is more scandalous than dropping the C bomb. You can air all of your dirty laundry in one Facebook status to the hundreds of people you're linked with, but you would never tell anyone your weight because *You Have Your Standards* and *That's a Personal Matter*.

Yes, the instinct is to feel embarrassed. I can feel the judge knocking at the door in my head. *Oi, fat cow. You really want to tell the world about this? Everyone's gonna picture you devouring everything in front of you, like a lion chewing on a deer carcass.* But I'm not embarrassed. I'm not letting the judge in this time, and I genuinely mean that.

Back then, I was going through a hard time. It was the extremes that led me to do it. The important thing is, I know I'm not a bad person for going through that.

Plus, I always replaced the bread. You can't take away a man's bread. That's just considerate!

If your instinct right now is to feel any kind of disgust at the scene I just described, I ask you to stop and take a couple of minutes to reflect. Try to empathise.

Is there anything in your life that you've been trying to get yourself to do for years? Maybe there's something you promise to change every New Year's Eve, but you always cave in? Are you disappointed with yourself when you don't do it? It could be something as simple as not managing to talk yourself into getting to the gym, or saving some money. You are not a bad person for failing. You're human. And most of the time, you don't even know what's stopping you from changing. All you know is that you constantly tell yourself off for it, and you have no idea why you just can't make yourself do it, you stupid cow. I assure you it's the same feeling. And the guilt and shame is even worse.

If you do feel any kind of judgement, or experience disgust at the scene that I just described, then I'm glad that I included it in my story. It's this kind of lack of understanding that I hope books like this can change.

Glossing over the low times, and making everything look pretty on the surface was what I tried to do for years, and it wasn't working.

CHAPTER 9

AGES OF YOU

I still remember vividly that night in Wetherspoons in 2013, on my birthday night out – when a horrible feeling of hopelessness descended upon me.

I was happy. I was laughing. I wanted to celebrate my 23rd birthday and my fab new figure in my beautiful flowery jump suit. I had cocktails in hand and I was surrounded by friends. I'd been dancing with people I loved and the night promised to be a good one. I was standing in a huge crowd of people and this time I wasn't worried that I was taking up more room than all of my friends combined. I felt hot as all hell, and not because I was sweaty.

So why did that sense of utter despair creep over me? Why did the panic grip my heart? Why did I ask myself 'what is the point?'

And more terrifyingly, why didn't I have an immediate answer for myself?

It scared me for days on end, until eventually I kind of forgot that it had happened. But only for a little while.

I mentioned that, as a young teen, I had a French pen pal. I also had a female pen pal for a short while. She wrote me a letter using a word I had never seen before – *déprimée*. I looked it up and to this day, I can still remember my heart sinking when I saw the meaning – *depressed*.

As a kid, I hadn't had any education on depression at all. So my first impression of reading it was that this person was going to be absolutely no fun to talk to! Why were they trying to be so different? Why couldn't they just cheer up? Shortly after that, my replies to her dwindled.

Now that I understand it more, I feel guilty. I wish, more than anything, that we'd had some education on mental illness as children. We learned about all other kinds of diseases in school – hell, even sexually transmitted ones. We all went to the dentist regularly, and we had regular check-ups at the doctors. What a different world it would be if children knew, from an early age, that they have nothing to feel ashamed about if they feel different or depressed? Maybe I wouldn't have been so dismissive of that French girl.

Now, though, I was just starting to wonder if I might be depressed. I had stopped seeing the point in anything. Often, I logically knew that I had had a good outing or had a nice time with friends or family, but I didn't actually feel the warm feeling that should have come with it. I stopped feeling passionate about my languages at all. They dried up completely. I went shopping one day and saw a necklace – it was very pretty, and I remember noticing that I *knew* that, but it didn't make me *feel* anything. I had stopped wearing jewellery a while before that, without even realising that I no longer wanted to make a top look that bit more pretty.

It wasn't something that I thought about all the time. It was just a thought that would visit me whenever my mind was idle, or when I felt I wasn't quite as happy with a situation as I should have been, like making social plans or doing something well at work. So, I entertained the idea, but always brushed it off; it wasn't something I understood at all.

Whenever I did hear about depression, it seemed a lot more serious, a lot graver than what I thought I was feeling myself.

Whenever I did give it some real thought, I would speak to other people who had it, or people who had lived with it. I would ask one simple question repeatedly:

'When you feel that way, is there a reason?'

I would always get an in-depth response, but it never really seemed to satisfy me – it didn't answer the question. Or, if I'm being completely honest with myself, it didn't give me the answer that I wanted to hear. Namely, I wanted to hear that depression came when you had a reason for it, and that if you fixed the initial problem, you would feel better. I had ideas in my mind of things that I wasn't happy with, and I was desperately hoping for someone to come along and say, 'Yes – this is what has made you depressed and this is what you do to get rid of it.'

But I never got that answer. And I know now that this is because depression doesn't always work that way. It is a lot more complex than that. The frustration that I used to feel when people couldn't say, 'Here, this is how you fix it …' was immense. But I never told anybody that I was asking for a reason. And I never said, 'Here are the reasons that I think I might be depressed – are they okay?' Perhaps that is what I should have said.

I think I also wanted to hear other peoples' reasons for their depression in case they were similar to mine – perhaps then I would have stopped telling myself that I was being silly. I would have told myself that it was okay to be depressed.

I didn't feel that I *deserved* to feel this bad about what was happening to me. It seemed petty. At the end of the day, I had a roof over my head, I had a family who loved me, I had a boyfriend, and lots of friends. What possible reason did I have to be depressed? I was constantly seeking the validation for how I was feeling. But since I wasn't being honest and telling people how I felt, there was only so much I could expect to get in return.

I'm reluctant to even use the word 'reasons' now, as I know that these problems were just as much, if not more, symptoms of my depression as they were reasons for it. But there were two main life-ruining themes that ran in my head every day, like a crap pop song that refused to go away.

(Just kidding, I love pop music. How *good* is Taylor Swift's 'Shake it Off?')

One – an obsession with aging and death

I had an unhealthy fixation with the notion of getting older. I was counting down the time in years and months until I was going to turn 30. I really don't know where this fixation came from – society? A passing comment made years ago? I may never know.

I would always have to count to the very month to make myself feel like I had that little extra bit of time. Some nights I would wake up with a jolt, heart racing, with a white-hot fear gripping my chest, the numbers running around my head. I would count forward, and then work out how long it had been since I had finished my degree … since I had left college … since I had left school. For all the fear it stirred up in me, I may as well have seen a ghost.

I don't think any of this was about death or mortality, it was more about my perceived lack of achievement.

However, a few months later, a family tragedy happened, and then I did have to deal with the reality of mortality. Mam's sister, auntie Elaine, developed lung cancer for the second time. The first time she got it, she had battled it with surgery and chemotherapy and had gone into remission. This time, she found out on Boxing Day that she had more tumours.

It was something I really felt I needed to talk about with my mother. Whenever she had news for us, Mam was very matter-of-fact about it. I don't think that she would have been comfortable if we thought she wasn't coping with it. She had to be the rock for her sister. I remember her being the same when Grandma passed away. Whenever I saw her cry about it, she would stop herself and reassure everyone around her that she was fine. She said she was just being silly. And she still does the same to this day. I don't know if this comes from upbringing, or from being a mother of five. All I knew at the time was that she was being unbelievably brave.

Eventually we found out that the cancer was terminal, and our auntie declined steadily after that. One time, I took my boyfriend with me to the pub to meet her and my mam. She was asking us about the house that we had just moved into together. I had recently gone full-time at the shop and talked my boyfriend into renting the place with me.) He'd wanted to wait, but I wasn't so patient. I had to start living life NOW! I couldn't wait to move out – I was getting older every day.

She was smiling at me, calling me darling, and I could feel her genuine happiness for me. I remember her face as clear as day in that moment, and I'll never forget it. I wasn't that close with her – but I felt a lot of love for her at that point.

We were all with her hours before we lost her. My mother's grief and the sadness of the whole situation was terrible. That's when my depression got steadily worse. But still I didn't tell anyone. There was actual, serious stuff going on. What right did I have to think of myself?

Secretly, I had developed a fear of chemicals in food. I was paranoid that I was going to give myself cancer by eating them. I refused to have artificial sweetener in my tea, opting instead to make myself drink unsweetened tea, or have sugar instead.

The fear of aging got steadily worse, and I was trying to research it to understand why it was happening. Why was I so scared?

None of the articles spoke to me, and I think it was because they weren't giving me a step-by-step guide on how to make the feelings go away. I wasn't interested in self-reflection or finding out why it was happening – I just wanted it gone so that I could look forward to my life instead of dreading it.

Two – an intense fear of change

I saw a saying once – probably a meme – that said, 'You can't start the next chapter of your life if you keep re-reading the last one.' Not only did I keep re-reading the last chapter, but I refused to even let go of the pages!

People in my life were moving on in all sorts of ways. That's a normal part of getting older. Some of the couples were breaking up, some were moving away, some were changing jobs, and some were making new friends. I told them all I was happy for them. I know I would have been a lot more supportive if I had been well.

It felt like the world I knew was disappearing in a tornado. As if it was picking up houses and people as it went, spinning them around me. Everything was moving way too fast, and I was standing dead still.

I replayed old memories constantly. It was upsetting that things had changed since then. I tried to see people as much as I used to, and resented people when they couldn't see me. Their lives were improving and it was exciting for them. But my life wasn't.

CHAPTER 10

FINAL STRAW

The summer of 2015 was when everything came tumbling down. I wasn't happy with any aspect of my life. I knew that. But still, I was safe in my comfort zone. (Better the devil you know.)

In May, I lost my job. The shop closed so I was made redundant. Even though it had been far from my dream job, it was still worrying financially.

I tried to save face, obviously. I told everyone that 'This Is A Good Opportunity'. (And in the end, it was.) I was going to do fantastic things and I was going to land myself a fantastic job. Or at least, that was my intention.

It's not what happened.

I lived in crippling fear the whole summer. My boyfriend would go to work every day in a job that he had recently started. It was extremely demanding and involved a lot of studying when he came home. I would stay at home, miserable during the day. I did everything I could to put off the job search, but I was determined to pay my way. I took all of my redundancy money and stretched it to the limit. And when that ran out, I took to selling my old "fat clothes" on eBay.

This served another purpose that helped me put off the job searching – it took up hours in the day. I would justify the time I spent at home by saying 'At least I'm making money!'

Stephanie brought full ring binders to the house, bursting with ideas for job searching, interviews and making speculative approaches to businesses. Then I would give her a reason why I could not do every single one of them, and it frustrated her so much because she just trying to help. Sometimes she'd try to ask me why I didn't feel like I could do any of the jobs, and I would have to ask her to stop talking. I wasn't trying to be rude, but I could feel panic and despair welling up in my chest when we discussed it and I didn't want to cry. And so our job sessions would just end in frustration.

I once read a book on how to become confident, written by a well-known hypnotist by the name of Paul McKenna. In it, he states that there is no such thing as having no confidence. He had spoken to many people who would swear up and down that they had no self-esteem and absolutely no confidence. When asked if they were absolutely sure, they had insisted they were. But, he pointed out, they did have confidence. They were completely confident in their opinion that they had no confidence!

That described me perfectly. I knew with a resounding certainty that I was useless, talentless, and had absolutely no foreign language skills whatsoever. I knew I would be pointed out as a fraud at any interview I would have the unbelievable luck to fall into. Try as she might, Stephanie could not change my mind. I had accepted it as a fact and that opinion just couldn't be changed.

It was soul-destroying and demeaning. I was a horrible person to be around. I didn't like me. My boyfriend didn't like me. I had no idea what my future held. My relationship was completely failing. We did nothing but argue. I took out every single bad mood on him and felt completely alone in my illness, while he struggled and eventually stopped trying to understand it. In the end, he stopped asking how I was. I hadn't asked him how he was for as long as I could remember.

Soon afterwards, we broke up. I had been in denial for a long time and still didn't expect it to happen, even though it needed to. In one summer, I lost my job, my house, my relationship, and the only vision of my future that I had known for the last six years. I was drowning in grief.

CHAPTER 11

BURNING HELL

There isn't a precise series of events in my head for the weeks that followed our breakup. In hindsight, I know when it was. I know how long the breakdown lasted. I can even tell you that this period lasted from the beginning of September 2015 through to at least the end of October, and then the depression lasted a while after that. I know I skipped both my dad's birthday and my friend's Halloween party to cry myself to sleep in bed. But I don't remember too well which bits happened when, and in which order.

I could barely face anybody. I didn't have a clue what was happening to me. I went to my mam's house, and I would stay there for months to come. I howled and cried myself to sleep. Mam was terrified of leaving me alone. I wasn't aware of drinking that much water, because I couldn't drink or eat a single thing from the second my crisis had started, but it must have come from somewhere, unless I'm some sort of secret camel. The first couple of days of crying probably made sense to everyone around me. After all, I'd had a rough few days. But when it started running into days four, five, and six ... you could see people were starting to get alarmed. I'd spent the entire week crying incessantly. My stepdad told my mother that he suspected a breakdown; he had never seen anything like it.

I Googled 'symptoms of a breakdown'. The consensus was that yes, crying for that length of time wasn't 'normal', or at the very least was something to be concerned about.

I must have tried to start a diary several times over – here is one entry I found in one of a million notebooks I had lying around:

This won't be structured like my usual diaries, I imagine. If I ever type it up to try to help someone someday, I'll try to find some order to it. Right now, I just need to get it out of me. *Just started on Prozac. I'm begging that this, alongside self-help, therapy, and meditating, is going to give me a fighting chance.*

And my current journey is a journey battling depression. I'm not talking winter blues or a down spell. I mean severe, don't-want-to-live, genuine physical pain in my heart and head depression. Feeling down was the starting station, depression is the railway and I'm hoping that the last stop is happiness and growth.

My aim is to get at least some of my dark thoughts onto paper so I can maybe take them out of my head long enough to sleep.

The breakup is the wound I'm nursing but the depression is the haemophilia that's stopping me even begin to heal. Anxiety is the salt rubbed in, and the obsessive thinking is continuing to rip the cut wider.

What's nice to see now is that even in the worst pain, I already knew that someday, I wanted to try to use my experience to help other people. Terri was still in there somewhere.

What's worrying is the fact that nothing follows this entry. The blank spaces that follow it mean much more to me than a few empty pages – they're menacing. They echo. What were the next few days like after writing that down? Who did I see? Which of my friends came to try to help me? Which of my family members' hearts did I break that week? Maybe all of them.

All I know is that at some point, after weeks of near complete isolation, my family and friends come to the rescue. I don't know when it happened, I don't know who talked to whom. All I know is that over the space of a few weeks, my fantastic, loving family and my unbelievable friends came together to form an army, helping me attack this illness on all fronts.

I'm a self-professed geek, but probably not in the most common sense of the word. I knit. I go to knitting groups and I go to wool festivals, and make happy noises when I see a beautifully dyed ball of silk or cashmere yarn. On payday, I treat myself to knitting and crochet tools, and I buy knitting magazines. I'm damn good at it too. In modern culture though, the 'geek' flag is waved high and proudly by gamers, readers and movie buffs.

I'm really quite uneducated when it comes to the different superhero storylines. But I do like *The Avengers*. Even though I know next to nothing about the backstory of the characters, I still rate it as one of my favourite films (which went down really well when I was being interviewed by my old boss for a job in the DVD shop). To me, the most hopeful and powerful image in any film I've seen is the moment when the Avengers are in the middle of the battle, and they come together (assemble, anyone?) in a circle to survey the scene unfolding around them. The Hulk roars. The others brandish their weapons. And they're the good guys, protecting people under attack.

What follows is the story of my breakdown, in as much detail as I can convey. But for every battle, I had a family member or a friend doing everything they could to help me fight.

As I think about it all now, I can picture an image of my friends, family and therapist, all coming to my rescue, like the Avengers, and it makes me giggle.

In my head, the film is called *Fuck You, Depression!* Here is the trailer. May contain spoilers.

CHAPTER 12

SO FAST, SO NUMB

As I said, I spent the first week straight crying non-stop, but the pain wasn't only emotional.

I was in the kitchen one day trying to cook sweet potato wedges and steak with my mother. We both knew I was unlikely to eat any of it, because my appetite had completely disappeared and I could barely choke down any food. But Mam knew how much I usually liked to cook, and I think she was trying to bring some normality back to my days. I hated those sweet potatoes at this point. Those solid bastards were really hard to cut with my mother's knife, and the glass chopping board kept shooting out from underneath me. The old me would have made a joke out of it, probably with some exaggerated fake tantrum. This time, I didn't. It was taking an unacceptable amount of my limited daily energy to turn this root vegetable into an acceptable shape to be called a wedge. The rest of my energy was going on pretending to be enjoying the whole experience so that my mother didn't worry. Ironically, the physical effort of making the whole meal would probably see me losing weight.

I took my 70th sip of water of the day. Mam looked at me strangely and asked what was wrong.

'I have something stuck in my throat, like I haven't got enough problems. I don't know what could be stuck though.'

I wrestled a bit more with the potatoes, and stared at the mushrooms browning like it was the most fascinating thing in the world. A few minutes passed and Mam piped up behind me.

'Apparently there's some muscle in the throat that can inflame when you're anxious,' she said, wielding her Samsung infused with the power of Google.

I read the article and didn't know whether I was relieved that I knew what it was, or devastated that it wasn't just something that I'd be able to flush away with a few Diet Cokes. It's called *globus hystericus* and there isn't actually anything stuck. But between that and the constant gripping pain around my heart, it was hard not to be terrified.

Headaches like I'd never experienced before often gripped me, and my only impulse was to pull my hair at the roots to distract me from the pain. Make no mistake, it gave me such lifted roots that I probably looked like a damn movie star (complete with a skinniness that can only come from a 600-calorie-a-day intake), but it didn't do a whole lot to make my family feel better.

On top of this, my mouth and tongue were completely numb. I couldn't feel my tongue on one whole side of my mouth, as if it had been burned with a hot drink.

Two days later, I went to Steph and her boyfriend's house, and they took me for a takeaway. It didn't matter how small my appetite was, they told me that I was going to eat something gross and greasy to get some calories into me, and I was going to enjoy every last bit. I promised to do it just for them. I didn't keep my promise.

I was completely unable to eat for several weeks into my breakdown. And I never did eat those potato wedges. The impulse to eat had just left my body. I kept drinking little sips of water to keep myself alive, but I wasn't finding joy in anything, and I didn't feel hungry because I was in too much pain. I was just too exhausted to register it. I wasn't feeling the natural instinct to eat that comes with hunger – I don't know if you have ever tried to eat when you are really, really not hungry, but believe me it is nearly impossible.

Let me reiterate: I absolutely love food. It is one of the biggest passions of my life. Whenever I plan a trip or a holiday, a lot of my priorities revolve around the meals I want and the restaurants I want to go to.

When I lived in Spain, my friends and I once packed our bags, went to the train station and chose a random city along the south coast to travel to. We found a local hostel, dropped off our bags, and after a sizzling and sunbathing ourselves on the beach, found a local restaurant and asked for the speciality of that region.

My friends did everything they could to try to make me eat. Bethan, my best friend from university, always made eating out ten times more fun, just by being there. Food excited her as much as it did me, especially Indian food, the only difference being that I was like the BFG and she was like a Polly Pocket – petite and blonde. She looked like a strong wind would carry her away. She came over to my house with our friend Sarah, and the two of them played me comedy films while putting Chinese takeaways under my nose, then watching me like a hawk to make sure I had taken at least a few bites.

My other close friend Matt and I have a common love of Italian food. We used to have regular 'pasta nights' where we would break open a couple of bottles of red wine and make pasta from scratch using a pasta maker that I'd bought him for his birthday. Matt was offended by my lack of appetite. His strategy was cheesecake.

He sat me down in the living room one day and placed a big slice of New York cheesecake down in front of us. He told me that he would only take a bite of his cheesecake whenever I ate a bite of mine. He was being theatrical and saying that he was really looking forward to the cheesecake, and that I was stopping him from eating it. I thought it was a good tactic; as a psychology graduate, he knew what he was doing.

There was only one friend that actually prevented me from eating. Lewis had managed to get me to agree to try some cereal, and gave me a bowl of Rice Krispies. A few minutes later I was eating my first and only mouthful when he made a joke that made me laugh so much I almost choked up. I didn't mind. He made me laugh more than anyone from the day I met him, and he didn't disappoint even now. That was the only time I can remember laughing throughout the breakdown.

Another time, my workmate Katie came to the house with an oversize birthday bag. It was full of things that were easy to eat or drink, and were full of calories to help fatten me up. Her boyfriend worked selling Lucozade to gyms and other places, so she brought me a range of flavours as well as energy bars and hot chocolates.

There was only one time in the day that I could bear to eat, and that was first thing in the morning. I knew I was frail and grey-skinned. I must have looked like a baby ostrich, considering how skinny and tall I was. I would take to the fridge and make the most of my momentary appetite by eating the fattiest things I could find for breakfast to bulk up my calorie intake for the day.

It took me a long time to agree to take any antidepressants. I know from hearing other people's stories that this reluctance often comes from embarrassment, or worrying what people will think. Too often, we struggle on, feeling the need to prove to everyone that we can cope without them. That wasn't the case for me. I was past the point of denying that I needed help, and I was severely mentally ill.

My reasons were different. Several friends and family members had told me over the years that for the first couple of months of taking antidepressants, you can actually become worse. For the simple reason that I couldn't comprehend the idea of getting any worse than I was, I 'knew' in my mind that there was no way I'd be able to take them.

When my family dragged me to the doctor the first time, he asked me if I believed I needed antidepressants. He assured me that they were not a one-stop fix-all solution – they would not make me happy. Rather, they would bring me to a solid, safe level for coping with my emotions, and this would be the foundation upon which I could start recovery.

I told him that I didn't think it was necessary.

'If I could just get some sleep,' I said to him, in between exhausted sobs, 'if I could just have something to help me sleep, to help me switch off for a few hours, I could be brave enough to face the day without antidepressants. Just please help me sleep.'

I could see the disappointment in my parents' eyes when I refused the antidepressants. And I knew why they were upset, but I had no way of conveying just how hard it was to get through the next ten minutes, never mind the thought that the pills could made me worse. In any case, they had to go along with my wishes.

A few weeks down the line, when I realised that sleeping pills weren't solving the problem, I eventually agreed to try the antidepressants. The doctor recommended a strong dose of Prozac, an antidepressant that can also be used to treat OCD.

From the depression side, I didn't experience any worsening symptoms. But when it came to anxiety, I was so much worse. I had a panic attack on a simple trip to the supermarket with my mother. It was the supermarket that my ex and I used to shop in all of time. There we were, in the dairy aisle, my mother seriously considering different yoghurt options before she would inevitably choose the exact same one as usual. She chose a flavoured yoghurt, and my eyes settles on the fat-free Greek style yoghurt. Every month I would buy a couple of pots of it for me and my boyfriend to have home-made coleslaw when we lived together. That small association was enough to trigger the anxiety attack.

I started to pace up and down the aisle, my breathing getting more and more shallow. I tried looking elsewhere, but everything I looked at was bringing back rapid flashbacks of the last time I was in there doing my own grocery shop. My chest squeezed impossibly tight and my ears started to ring; I asked my mother to give me the car keys and I spent the rest of the hour in tears in the car while my poor mother had to finish her shop. Adele played on the radio. I wanted to throw it out of the window.

Another time, I gave myself the goal of going to the central library. It was a long walk and then, once I was there, I knew that I wouldn't sit and cry because I would be in public. Halfway there, I had the biggest and worst panic attack I had ever had. My entire body was throbbing in pain from the headache and my rapid heart rate. I felt like my breath was caught in my throat. I remember standing in the middle of the street and looking both ways around me – and realising that either way, I was nowhere near home and couldn't get to privacy any time in the next few minutes.

I knew, though, that I couldn't go the library and so I chose to walk home, tears streaming down my face the whole time. I'd honestly thought I was about to achieve something that was (to me, at least) massive, but I wasn't even strong enough to do that. Getting up to go the library had been an absolutely massive step for me – my biggest previous achievements had been getting dressed and getting to the bottom of the stairs by myself.

For a long time after that, I struggled to go into any retail space, especially large shopping centres.

CHAPTER 13

SECOND GUESSING

Me and my triplet sisters always had slightly addictive / obsessive personalities. Growing up, if the three of us found a hobby, we would become pretty much addicted to it. We all had some odd fixations and collections in our isolated lives. On the nights that we would sit at home in our rooms while the other kids went out, we would sit and apply ourselves to whatever new game, craft, hobby, TV show, or gimmick we'd grown addicted to that month.

I was hooked on keeping diaries. I bought them in all styles, sizes, and layouts. I wrote a record of every single day as and when it happened. At the same time, Toni found a new obsession for painting – she covered every wall of her bedroom from floor to ceiling with her creations. Stephanie was a collector of fountain pens, books, and even at one point, money. She would count it out every night like someone out of *A Christmas Carol*. As I got older, I started hoarding craft items, and I would knit any spare minute I got. That was helpful, cathartic even. But, as things got worse, even my worrying started to feel obsessive.

It seems to make sense to me, then, that one of the symptoms of my breakdown would be obsessive rumination. I had lived through worry before, but this was a different beast altogether. As explained by Dr. Bruce Hubbard, unhealthy worry is your mind's preoccupation with fear of the future and perceived threats to come. Whenever I worried in the past, I could be reassured to some extent that everything was going to be okay, or I could reason with myself that I could change the outcome of a situation if I was brave enough.

Obsessive rumination, however, is a complete and total inability to stop an endless damaging cycling of distressing thoughts pertaining to your past. I couldn't stop myself from replaying painful memories and I didn't stand a chance against the never-ending onslaught of self-torture about all of the things I had done wrong in the last few years.

The pure trauma of the rumination is why I've developed a pet peeve for people using the term 'OCD' to talk about themselves liking to be tidy, or clean, or neat and in control. Even though I can appreciate the meaning behind it, it makes me cringe. I have read that obsessive rumination is one of the extreme symptoms of obsessive compulsive disorder, and I only struggled with it for a few months. If I had to live a whole lifetime with obsessive rumination to the degree that I had it, I'm not sure where I would be right now. I take my hat off to anyone who has overcome similar symptoms. I think it was the hardest part for my family.

From my sisters' point of view, it seemed like my mind was running non-stop and I was completely unable to switch it off. I was desperately trying to find something of hope or sense to cling onto, and it led me to ask questions over and over – often the same ones – repeated tens of times. As soon as I accepted an answer, my mind would seem to go over whatever evidence it had to the contrary and broke down again, so there was no stability to my mindset. I know it was really hard for my sisters: I looked exhausted mentally and physically, and I looked weak. I went to sleep sobbing and woke up sobbing, and I continued the obsessive questioning. The questions covered everything, from whether it was my fault that my relationship had ended, through to whether it was possible to ever be happy again. Or was I really losing it? Would I be sent to hospital?

They desperately wanted to give me some peace but were terrified of making promises to me in case they turned out not to be true. So they were constantly choosing between helping me get through the next five minutes and avoiding disappointment further down the line. They told me that, being triplets, my pain felt like theirs, and it was ridiculously painful to see me struggling so much without being able to take it all away. I was exhausted and needed more than anything for my mind to give me a rest, but it wasn't happening. I didn't have any energy to recover.

It was also a huge test on their patience. There were only so many times a day that my parents or sisters could repeat the same information to me. Every now and again, tears would fill their eyes, they would lose it, and snap or shout at me to get a grip on myself, and stop doing what I was doing. But I couldn't. I felt like I was on factory reset every few minutes. One minute, somebody could convince me it wasn't my fault that my life was falling to hell. But within five minutes, my poorly mind had dragged up a million hurtful images to prove me wrong, rational or otherwise.

Remember the time you were in a bad mood and screamed at your boyfriend for no reason? You don't deserve to be loved.

Remember the time you wished you had another job? You jinxed it. You're the reason you lost it all.

Toni had taken some counselling from the NHS when she was younger and had been given some cognitive behavioural therapy (CBT). It was a therapy based on identifying harmful ways of thinking and behaving, caused by anxiety and depression, and then providing coping strategies based on rational and evidence-based thinking. She showed me something called 'If and then statements'. The idea is that you write down whatever the nasty thought is, and then write down the opposite, more positive, thought and the evidence for it right beside it. IF I had the nasty thought, THEN I should remember the kinder one. She gave me a Winnie the Pooh notebook and told me to carry it with me. She wrote down the first ones, and handed it over to me with hope in her eyes. The problem was that I couldn't concentrate for long enough to write them down – if I was mid-sentence, I would have to stop and ask them the question all over again.

Thank heavens the Prozac (OCD antidepressants) eventually started to kick in, because the whole thing was mental torture for me and incredibly frustrating and distressing for everyone else. Slowly but surely my obsessive thoughts began to subside a little, and I felt the first bit of hope that I could one day jump off the spinning hamster wheel for good. The more I was able to let go of the grip that the thought cycle had me in, the more I could focus on trying to make myself do every day normal things, like get out bed and leave the house.

Happiness was still a speck of dust on the horizon at the moment, but hope was emerging.

CHAPTER 14

MAKE IT ALL OKAY

Mam told me she could see the turning point; after a while, it became clear that all I wanted was to get better.

I hurt and scared my family so many times by telling them that I couldn't take it anymore. Make no mistake about it, I meant it. I had absolutely no idea how I was going to make it through the next five minutes, but there were also two emotions still inside me that wouldn't, and couldn't, go away. One was my love for my family. The second was the need to get better. These emotions weren't strong, raging fires that I felt passionately. I didn't have any strength for that. They were more like anchors: solid and strong, and they kept me in place. Yes, I wanted out of the hell, but I wanted to do it by finding happiness again.

I'm aware of how lucky I am that I never got to the point of giving up completely, though. What a lot of people don't understand – what I don't expect anyone who hasn't experienced it to understand – is that not wanting to be alive, and wanting to die are two different things. I didn't want to die. I wasn't going to do anything to hurt myself. But I did wish that I had never been born. Being alive, and conscious, and constantly aware of the pain – simply being unable to ever switch off – was terrifying and agonising.

Toni and Stephanie, in their heartbreak, were doing everything they possibly could to help pull me through. My little bookworm, Stephanie, went shopping with our dad and they brought me back a Kindle. I remember I was happy about it, or at least knew that I should be happy. At the very least, I was really grateful. They bought me every single book that Steph thought could help me and loaded the Kindle up, so that even when they were at work and couldn't be there to do anything, I had something to help.

Some of them worked well, long-term. One, though, had such a negative impact on me that I feel sick when I remember it. Mam was on holiday. I had convinced Dad that I would be alright sleeping at the house by myself because Steph was going to come around and make sure that I was settled, fed and bathed before she drove back home. In my pyjamas, I got tucked into bed with a sugary cup of warm milk (to help me sleep and to get some calories into my system). Stephanie gave me a kiss and set off home. She asked me if I wanted her to stay, but I told her not to. I picked up my Kindle and started to read.

It was written by somebody who had recovered from severe depression and so I knew that somewhere in the book, they were going to reveal their recovery techniques. That was the real reason I was reading it. *Come on, tell me now what I need to do to get better so that I can start doing it now!* What I didn't anticipate was how many chapters of despair I was going to have to read through to get to it.

After reading one scene in which the author described, in detail, being unable to get out of bed, I began to have a panic attack. They had gone through the sort of things that I had experienced over the last few weeks, and the stories weren't getting easier, they were getting worse.

I couldn't handle it. I saw white spots in my vision and my chest contracted. I let out the same primal howl that I had let out on that first night of my breakdown, right here in the same bed in my mam's house, and through the sobs, I started to beg my empty room:

'Please help me. I don't want to do this anymore.'

When I had calmed down a couple of hours later, after already having messaged Toni and caused Steph to jump right back in her car and drive back to Hull, I deleted the book.

I was hearing more than enough from every Tom, Dick and Harry that I would come out of this stronger, and that I just needed to give it time. They told me I was going to get better. Even though I know in hindsight that every word of it was true, even though I know there is sometimes very little you can say in that situation to make someone feel better, I still wanted to punch anyone who talked like that to me.

What good were those words to me? How did they help me? I didn't need meaningless soundbites. I needed someone to tell me right now, what the hell I needed to actually *do* to get better. Someone out there was going to be helped massively by this book. I knew that. It was going to change lives. But I wasn't ready for it yet. I wanted a practical manual, a how-to-recover guide, and I needed it now.

I was reminded of when I was 21. I needed a dress for the university ball, and went into my favourite shop (and by favourite, I mean one of the only shops left that sold nice clothes for women of my stature, that of a double decker bus). I headed for the brightly coloured ones to complement my blazing red hair. I felt I needed to avoid block colours or (shock, horror) white. I didn't want to look like a cherry bakewell cake.

A beautiful dress, bright blue at the top with lace and a black skirt, called out to me. I tried on the size 22 and it was too binding. Picking up a size 24, I realised that having a clothes size higher than your age, post-puberty, was shocking. It was a wakeup call to stop saying 'When I lose the weight ...' and actually lose the damn weight.

At that time, there were advertisements everywhere for another of Paul McKenna's books, claiming to help you lose weight by hypnotising your mind into believing that you had a gastric band fitted. I wasn't after a quick fix; I had six stone to lose. If I did it by crash dieting, I was just going to end up looking like one of those shrivelled up balloons you find in the corner after a child's birthday party. Exercise wasn't a problem, I loved swimming and badminton and could even hack the cross-trainer if I was feeling particularly masochistic. But my relationship with food and the psychology of it all was a much bigger challenge, so I felt like it was worth a try.

Long story short, by the time my 21st birthday had rolled around, I had lost three stone. The book was working. The man was a genius.

So, knowing my past success with his books, Steph bought me *I Can Mend Your Broken Heart*, and Toni bought me *I Can Make You Happy*. Whether you believe in the premise of the hypnosis or not, it cannot be denied that the man has some eye-opening psychological insights and explanations for the sort of problems we have all been slaves to at some point in our lives.

A fascination for reading about psychology and understanding what on earth was happening to me was born. I was not interested in sitting around and waiting for the magical healing that everyone was always telling me that time would bring. After all, if your car is broken, you don't sit around waiting for it to mend. You need to find out what the problem is, how to fix it, and what caused it to begin with. That way, you can prevent it from happening again.

CHAPTER 15

I WALKED WITH A ZOMBIE

One of the biggest worries for my family was that I was by myself a lot at home while everyone else was at work. Stephanie was working in Bradford at the time, and Toni had moved to Leeds for her job. My big sisters both worked too, and when they weren't at work, they were looking after my nieces and nephews. My mam and stepdad looked after me whenever they could, but they had jobs to go to as well. So, for a few hours a day at least, I had to cope with my crisis alone.

Friends and family continued to check in on me throughout the day. Sometimes I'd be honest and tell them I wasn't really coping, wasn't really sleeping, and was struggling to get out of bed and shower. But then, of course, that would really make them panic. Sometimes I just didn't want to burden people and I told them I was 'fine'. But fine for me was just managing to get from one hour to the next.

Dad worked full-time too, but he had a lot of annual leave saved up at his job, and he started taking some half days off from work to come and be with me. We wouldn't do anything fancy – we would just walk.

There's a small town that kind of attaches itself to the edge of Hull, called Hessle. The Humber Bridge is on Hessle Foreshaw and stretches across the River Humber. We would take walks over the bridge or through the parks surrounding it. It was peaceful and felt like a bit of an escape from my life, which seemed to be falling apart around me.

The first few times he did this it must have felt like walking around with a zombie. I was drawn, skinny, grey, and quiet. I would just stare into the distance. Dad is one of the quieter ones in our family, but he talked away to me, talking about things to distract me or asking me how I was feeling.

Most of the time I just concentrated on putting one foot in front of the other. I would answer my dad, often in one word or short sentences. But even that was enough. It was important for me to get out of the house anyway.

The more we went walking, the closer I felt to Dad. When I found myself more able to speak, I would open up to him about things I'd never really talked to him about before. We'd also talk about more light or trivial things, and it did help. It didn't solve anything, but it was far better than wallowing in my own misery at home.

I'm sure there's a lot of studies that look at the physical benefits of walking with depression, and I reckon there'll be evidence to suggest it really helps lift your mood. But for me the benefit was more in the therapeutic aspects of it. I started to notice that I enjoyed cool breezes and the sound the breeze made when it flowed through the trees. I liked that I couldn't hear lots of cars and people talking.

Every breath I took and every thought I had still hurt me, but being able to talk to Dad – when I was in the right head space for it – served as a form of talking therapy. Perhaps that was when I started to realise the power of talking in trying to get better.

CHAPTER 16

RAPID EYE MOVEMENT

A couple of months into my breakdown, I told Stephanie that I was ready for a therapist. She'd been asking me to go and see one for a while but I hadn't had the strength to even think about it. But now, I was ready.

Steph was delighted. She whipped out the information she'd found on a local therapist – ever prepared to help me. She'd called him up and asked if he could help. 'We don't have a lot of money,' she'd told him, 'but me, my sisters, and my parents are all willing to chip in for sessions, as she's lost her job. Just please help us. We're desperate.'

As it turned out, Peter had a free spot available for emergency situations and he agreed to see me as soon as possible.

Stephanie booked in a session and drove into Hull to take me in.

The office was at the end of a stunning garden, at the bottom of a lane that snaked through blooming flowers and ponds. From inside, you could hear the sound of wind-chimes and a water fountain. With this, the ambient lighting and warmth inside made it a very tranquil and safe-feeling space.

Peter was extremely approachable, everything I could have asked for in a therapist. He was gentle and considerate and put me at ease immediately.

The first few weeks involved talking therapy. I talked and talked and talked about who I was, my past and what had happened to me. It was weeks before I went into a session and didn't cry all the way through.

Peter assured me there was nothing wrong with me, that I had had a very tough few years and the events of the current year had been one too many and had pushed me into a pit. The job ahead of us was to bring myself out of it and then, once I had a firm footing, build a happier future.

He often stopped me when I would be on a self-criticising rant. He told me that the negative things I said about myself was the voice of the judge, a nasty, unhelpful inner monologue that told me I was worthless, just like the years of bullying. It was hard not to picture Judge Judy.

Talking about my depression and my life leading up to it was just the kind of catharsis I needed. When I finally started having any real length of time between tears and there was nothing else to recount, we started to discuss what techniques we were going to use in the coming months. Peter was a fully trained expert in a therapy called EMDR that I had never heard of personally.

I can't give a better outline of the therapy than the one given by the EMDR Association on their website:

'EMDR is an acronym for 'Eye Movement Desensitisation and Reprocessing'. EMDR is a powerful psychological treatment method that was developed by an American clinical psychologist, Dr Francine Shapiro, in the 1980s.[2]

When a person is involved in a distressing event, they may feel overwhelmed and their brain may be unable to process the information like a normal memory. The distressing memory seems to become frozen on a neurological level. When a person recalls the distressing memory,

2 http://emdrassociation.org.uk/whatis-emdr/

the person can re-experience what they saw, heard, smelt, tasted or felt, and this can be quite intense. Sometimes the memories are so distressing, the person tries to avoid thinking about the distressing event to avoid experiencing the distressing feelings.

Some find that the distressing memories come to mind when something reminds them of the distressing event, or sometimes the memories just seem to just pop into mind. The alternating left-right stimulation of the brain with eye movements, sounds or taps during EMDR, seems to stimulate the frozen or blocked information processing system.

In the process the distressing memories seem to lose their intensity, so that the memories are less distressing and seem more like 'ordinary' memories. The effect is believed to be similar to that which occurs naturally during REM sleep (Rapid Eye Movement) when your eyes rapidly move from side to side. EMDR helps reduce the distress of all the different kinds of memories, whether it was what you saw, heard, smelt, tasted, felt or thought.'

It sounded to me like a good theory, and I was ready to try it. My rapid eye movement was guided by a small machine that I held in my hand with two hand-pieces that lit up alternately. Peter gave me an iPod with some serenity and tranquillity music that would play lightly in my ears, but low enough that I could still hear us talking above it.

We would 'prep', ready for the session. Peter would start by asking me what it was that I wanted to work on. Most of my choices revolved around early bullying memories that still haunted me. But I also addressed issues that had been caused by the breakdown itself. Here, I will use the example of my anxiety around my mobile phone, i.e. I was finding it difficult to answer a call or open a text message without fear, my heart racing or ignoring the text for a couple of days.

I was asked to think of the earliest possible memory I had of this happening. I gave the memory of when I first had my breakdown and being too scared to look at my phone because the messages from family or friends, asking me to explain how I was, were too hard to face.

I was asked to rate on a scale of 1–10 how distressing the memory was.

I was asked to give a negative thought or belief that I had about myself as a result of this memory. I told him that I believed that when I answered the call, it would be something upsetting or about something that I had done wrong.

I was then asked what thought or belief I wanted to hold about myself instead. I told him that I wanted to believe that I was in control, even if the message or call was something unpleasant.

I was asked to rate on a scale of 1–7 how true I currently believed that to be. He made a note of each, and then began the lights, asking me to replay the memory as vividly as I could while watching them.

Sometimes I felt that I wasn't doing it right if my mind would stray from the original memory and onto other similar instances. I told Peter as such and he assured me I should go with it. In intervals of around half a minute each, Peter would stop the lights and ask me 'What was happening'. I found this an interesting way of asking how I was, but it steered me to explain to him what my thought processes were, rather than just declaring that I was 'okay' or 'not okay'.

It didn't feel real at first and I felt sceptical. There were moments where I felt silly. When he asked what was happening, I would sometimes go quiet while I tried to think of what the 'right' answer should be.

Sometimes, I would keep playing the memory until it just stopped having any impact. For others, I would be struck with the determination to go out and do something brave after the session, like make a scary phone call or read through all my emails that I currently had buried.

At the end of each session, I was asked the same questions that I had been given before the process started. The aim was to feel no distress when thinking about the memory anymore. Some of the more distressing memories could take two or more EMDR sessions to clear. They were draining and I was always told that I could stop absolutely whenever I wanted to. If any epiphanies or changes in emotions happened, which happened a lot, we discussed them at length.

There are memories that Peter and I 'processed' now that I am able to talk about matter-of-factly, without the punch in the stomach or stab to the heart feeling they used to have. Sceptics would argue that this is through talking the matter through – but all I can say is that simply talking about them in the past had never had this profound an effect in this short a timeframe. EMDR worked, and it was incredibly powerful.

CHAPTER 17

I DON'T SLEEP, I DREAM

If I had to choose which of the physical symptoms of the breakdown is the worst, insomnia would win by a landslide. Sleep has always been something I've been able to do easily. There is no sweeter feeling than knowing that, after a long week at work, I have a lie-in waiting for me on a Saturday morning. Almost nothing can compare to the pure happiness of waking up at what feels like 6.00am, looking at my alarm clock and seeing 1.00 am staring right back at me. Even if I wake up an hour before I have to get up for work, I can fall back to sleep instantly.

But that was all taken away from me. The first night of my breakup and break*down*, I woke up in a jolt, unable to catch my breath for a few moments as a heavy crushing pain landed on top of me. I thought I must have had at least six hours. The previous day felt like weeks ago. I looked at my phone, and it said 12.00. It'd been even longer than I thought. I tried to sit up and that's when I realised that it was dark behind the pale-yellow curtains. Behind the ringing in my head, I was confused. Was it raining outside? Even England doesn't get that gloomy in summer. And then I realised it had been an hour. One hour of sleep, and it felt like weeks. I knew that there were other people in the house trying to sleep, but I couldn't stop the howl of pain that came out. It was completely involuntary.

I lost around two stone in the first week and a half of my breakdown. And while a large part of that was due to the fact that I couldn't force food down, I genuinely believe that some of it was down to the hours of incessant moving around in the night, willing myself to fall asleep, hoping to catch a few precious hours of oblivion. It didn't happen; it was impossible. My head hurt, my chest was in a vice. My throat was almost closed from crying.

The dark was terrifying. There was nothing here except me, a bed, and my thoughts. Obsessive. Incessant. Painful. And the promise of a stretch of hours in front of me that wouldn't end. So, I tried to turn on the lights to scare some of the thoughts away. But this posed another problem; the glowing strip of light that came through the bottom of the door was a menacing signal in the middle of the night that I wasn't resting.

My memory of it is hazy now, but at some point I had managed to get some sleeping pills from the doctor. I can't remember what they were called. But for some reason I had such an adverse reaction to them – I began hallucinating and telling my family that I no longer wanted to live – that Stephanie and my mam had to take me to A&E. I stopped taking them straight away and fell back into my pattern of sleeplessness.

Each morning after that, Mam could tell me what time I was awake and for how long. I managed to feel a twinge of guilt through the pain and tried to make a mental note not to use the light the next night, so that she could get up for a drink or go to the bathroom in the night without worrying that I was on the other side of the door, crying alone instead of sleeping. I didn't manage to stick to this new plan by the time the next night came around. That decision was 12 hours ago. A lifetime ago. A time I barely remembered.

So, Mam's research began. She was Supermother and Google was her trusted sidekick. One day, early on, she came home with candles, muscle relaxing bubble bath, malt biscuits, a lava lamp, and an extra couple of bottles of milk. At 8.00 pm, she drew me a bath, lit candles around it and turned the light off. She handed me an iPod that Stephanie had given her, which had hours upon hours of radio time and podcasts featuring Steven Merchant, Ricky Gervais, and Karl Pilkington. She told me to take a bath and listen to something funny. It will rest my eyes, distract me, and make me feel calm, she said.

I did as she said. When I came out, she could hear me. Even when she left me alone to give me some space, she could tell from my footsteps where I was in the house. Meerkat Mother. Within a few minutes of me changing into my pyjamas and climbing into bed, she had come upstairs, a mug of warm milk in one hand and exactly three malt biscuits in the other (she knew I could only eat two, so she kept trying to convince me to eat three. Mostly it was just really handy for whenever there was a biscuit-falling-in-the-drink related casualty).

She pointed to the end of the room where the lava lamp was glowing in the corner. She told me to watch it for a while if I didn't want to close my eyes, and try to clear my mind as much as possible. 'It's pretty,' she said, 'and it's meant to be really relaxing.'

It started to work, and for a couple of those hours, it was a deep, restful sleep.

I couldn't relax for long, however. Once my body had got used to getting some sleep, my mind was finally able to kick into gear.

I've never been able to watch horror films. My sisters and I have a best friend who has been in our lives since we were about four years old. We spent every day together at school, playing, joking, occasionally fighting, but always together. We loved, and still love, the heck out of him. I remember laughing at almost everything he said. He always had something exciting, like this fun new game on his computer called *The Sims*, or one of those pencil cases that has buttons you could press to make a pencil sharpener, or a ruler, or an eraser pop out of a secret compartment.

I remember once when we were in our early teens, the age where a lot of kids start watching horror films. A film called *Ghost Ship* came out in 2002, and we must have been 13 or 14 by the time we got around to watching it. It was the weekend and we were staying with Dad as usual, and he came round to see us with the DVD of *Ghost Ship* in hand.

I already knew at that point that I couldn't handle seeing anything bloody or tense. As a small kid I had one of those Funfax diaries, and there was a section in it where you had to fill out cute little 'facts' about yourself:

What is your favourite colour? Red.

What is your favourite book? Twin Trouble by Ann M. Martin.

(I had bought it along with the Funfax at the school book fair, because it was about twins and one of them was called Terri. My young self was really amused by that).

What scares you? James Bond, because I don't like shooting.

(I had accidently seen a family member watching James Bond when I was really small, and the sight of someone being shot had shaken me to my core for years).

But for whatever reason, we all sat and watched *Ghost Ship*. The ghostly aspects were creepy enough. And then came a scene where everyone in a vast ballroom on the ghost ship gets sliced apart by razor wire. There was blood everywhere and people were trying to hold onto their sliced limbs and grab onto each other. I remember feeling sick and shaking, and not sleeping great for a few days after that. Even writing about it now, my stomach is churning.

I stayed away from horror films after that, and to this day, I do not watch them. I won't even entertain the idea of getting used to them. I'm squeamish around blood and scenes of violence and pain, especially shootings and stabbings.

Because I've never let myself watch anything violent, my 'bad dreams' growing up were always about some sort of extreme stress or threat instead. They didn't happen all that often, but it was always a rotation of the same few dreams. There was the tooth-loss dream ...

My teeth are becoming looser and looser, one by one. I'm trying to keep them in my mouth and hide the problem from everyone else. Sometimes my jaw locks shut, and I try my hardest to open my mouth, but I know it's making my teeth crack and chip.

And then there's the dream when I'm in school again ...

I'm trying to get to my history class, and I'm going around and around the second floor, trying to find the classroom. But no matter what I do, or how many times I complete a lap of the school, I can't find it. I know it's close by, and I know it's with my favourite teacher. The stress is building – my exams are in two weeks and I have already missed the last eight classes because I couldn't find the room the last few weeks either. I am going to fail my exam.

Now, though, I really knew what bad dreams are. A few weeks into the breakdown, I started to get some sleep. And by this, I mean that for one or two hours a night, my body switched off through pure exhaustion. But I woke up in a horrible way every single night.

The first time it happened was one of the most surreal things I had ever experienced. We've all seen films where the main character is having a disturbing dream, the music builds to an ominous crescendo, and they sit bolt upright in bed, hair perfectly brushed, make up flawless. It was similar for me, except when I jolted upright, I looked like I'd just been electrocuted after being dragged backwards through a hedge after a night of heavy drinking! In the seconds that followed, my brain tried to work out what had happened. My heart was thumping at a mile a minute, I could barely breathe and vivid images from my dreams raced through my head.

I may have finally been getting some semblance of sleep, but it was nothing like the oblivion I'd been hoping for. The dreams – that's actually too nice a word – the *nightmares* – were violent, bloody, sickening ...

I am being chased by a poisonous gas. It's a pearly white mist and I'm running through a hallway made up of nothing but large, white, jagged bricks on the wall. The floor is made of a smooth marble that's hard to run on, and wet. I need to get away from the gas. Nobody has told me what it is, or what it will do if I breathe it in, but I do know with a frightening clarity that I can't let it get anywhere near me. I finally escape the building through an emergency door, but the gas retains its density and continues to pursue me like a beast. It's slow moving and without urgency, but this doesn't reassure me. It's like it has a mind of its own and knows it will catch up anyway, no matter how fast I run away from it.

I reach a cliffside now; the only way is up. I'm a terrible climber. The rocks are cutting my hands and the blood is making my grip slippery. The gas is at my feet. Right as I'm about to reach the top of the cliff, my point of view changes and I'm looking down at myself from the clifftop. I look like I did when I was 17 – slight and blonde, young and vulnerable. A horrific, blood-curdling, gargling scream starts and I know I've been caught.

And Ewan McGregor is there. I don't know what that's about!

One night in early October, my mother and her husband had gone on holiday and I had the house to myself. She was really worried about my being there alone, to the point that she almost cancelled her holiday. But she'd had this trip planned for a long time, and she was exhausted, just like every one of my family members. She would spend her days at work, worried sick, and then came home to look after the ghost of her daughter. My sisters and I convinced her not to cancel – my dad was just around the corner he would be there to look after me.

I had a friend who called herself Wolfie. Whenever I was feeling particularly distressed, I reached out to her. She struggled with mental health issues for most of her adult life and has learned a lot along the way. She was always open and honest about it with me, which I found really admirable, since I now know how much depression can make you feel ashamed and embarrassed.

And so, the night my mother was away, it seemed only logical that she was the person I texted. My message read:

'Please. Please tell me this is going to end soon. I can't take it anymore.'

Within 15 minutes, she was standing at my door. I didn't have the room in my head for any more emotions, but she held me and told me she understood exactly how I was feeling. She said, 'It can, and will, get better.' I didn't have many words in me, so mostly I just rocked in her arms and cried.

Eventually I found my voice and I kept asking her how long it was going to take. I didn't know if I could keep going much longer.

A small while later, I heard the sound of a key in the lock, and Steph walked in. Wolfie looked at me sheepishly and admitted that she had sent her a text asking her to come over. I suppose that, to her, the situation must have looked quite extreme, and merited something drastic Steph driving down from Goole. In reality, although I could see it breaking her heart all over again, this was nothing unusual for Steph. I had been this way for a few months now and Steph had been looking after me a lot.

I told them both about the insomnia and explained that I hadn't had anything to help me sleep since the demon sleeping tablets I'd had from the doctor. I'd been too scared to take anything since.

'Enough's enough. There has to be something else you can take. Let's go the pharmacy and ask them if there is anything over the counter that can help you. Even if it's herbal,' Stephanie said.

They put me into a car and we drove to a nearby pharmacy. On the way, Wolfie told us about some of her experiences and some of the things that helped her. She told us that one of her coping strategies was to picture the Hulk looking after her. He would stand in front of her, protecting her from whatever was causing her distress. A true protector. I really liked that idea.

I was so exhausted that the sheer act of putting on shoes and leaving the house left me with heavy limbs. Talking was almost impossible. I wished I'd been able to tell Wolfie that what she said cut through some of the fog and hit home. Instead, I nodded slightly and let Steph do all the talking.

Later on, I mentioned the nightmares to my therapist, Peter. I told him that they stayed with me for days afterwards, replaying in my head and, if anything, they were becoming sharper and more vivid as time passed. Visualisation is a powerful thing – when it comes to anxiety, your mind often cannot tell the difference between an imagined threat and a real one, which explains why a person's heart will race with adrenaline at the thought of something super stressful. He told me that sometimes, a good way to deal with nightmares, if the images won't go away, is to re-imagine them over and over again with something different happening – something funny – until they no longer pose a threat.

Although not a particularly original trait of mine, one of my favourite books is Harry Potter. In the third book, there is a magical creature called a bogart, which is essentially a shapeshifter that takes on the form of whatever scares you the most. Neville Longbottom, the geeky kid, is terrified of the potions master, Snape, and so the bogart takes Snape's form whenever it is around Neville. The Defence Against the Dark Arts teacher tells the student to think of something funny, and they learn to perform a spell which adds that funny quality to whatever scary form the bogart takes. Neville imagines Snape wearing his grandmother's clothes, and suddenly it isn't scary anymore. What Peter was suggesting to me was something along those lines.

I told Peter what Wolfie had said about the Hulk. He smiled and said, 'Do you think that you have anyone similar that you can use who can be your 'protector'?'

I thought for a few minutes. 'Not really … but I don't see why the Hulk wouldn't work. There's a funny moment in the Avengers film where he has a tantrum and throws the bad guy around like a ragdoll.'

In my head, the Hulk emerged from the middle of a pearly white mist. He manages to grab a hold of it, and he throws it around, slamming it into the ground and roaring.

The Hulk stayed with me for months after that. I even used him as a phone wallpaper for a while. Long after I started getting more sleep, long after the anxiety nightmares calmed down, he was still there. It worked for bad memories, too. I brought him in to beat the hell out of anyone in my mind that had done something bad. And slowly, over time, they stopped bothering me. And all from a passing comment made by a friend who was trying to pick me up during a tough time. The accidental hero.

CHAPTER 18

WHY NOT SMILE

A recent annual health survey in England showed that 19% of people believed mental health issues are partly a matter of people having no self-discipline or willpower.

I had five different doctors over the space of my recovery from depression, not including Peter, my psychotherapist. I spoke to them about medication, counselling, and the physical symptoms of depression.

On one of my trips to the doctor, I told him that I had been suffering with depression, that I'd been taking medication for it, and I was there for a catch up. I wanted to know if my dosage needed changing, and if I still needed a sick note, or if it was time for me to start job searching. The doctor, a man I hadn't seen before, turned away from the screen and looked at me thoughtfully.

'Do you know that last week I had a 16-year-old girl here who needed a hip replacement?'

'Right ...?'

'And we also have a teenage girl who has cancer.'

'That's terrible.'

I just looked at him for a few seconds, waiting for the actual point.

Crickets chirped in my head; if tumbleweed had blown across the room I wouldn't have been surprised. He continued to look at me, waiting for whatever point he was making to suddenly hit me like an epiphany.

'What I'm saying is … there are people who come in here with actual problems.'

The shock was instantaneous. My cheeks flamed, the stunned laughter came out. I took the next few seconds to work up a good rage. I had just experienced the worst four months of my fucking life. I had cut out almost everyone I knew because I was so embarrassed about what I was going through. It had taken every bit of energy I had to open up about my issues. I was fighting to make my own body do everyday things to help me function normally, and this man was telling me that I didn't have a 'real' problem.

'I think that's a really dangerous thing for a man in your position and with your responsibility to say,' I said to him, my eyes locked straight onto his. 'That's a really insulting attitude and that's what makes people keep it a secret in the first place. If I wasn't so embarrassed about it and worried that people wouldn't understand, I would have got help for this years before it ever got this far. I never claimed to be as bad as someone with cancer, but I absolutely do have a problem and I deserve to get help for it without being made to feel like I'm being silly. I'm one of the lucky ones because I'm recovering, but this disease actually claims lives.'

The doctor took a sharp intake of breath and went slightly red.

Suddenly, his tone was softer and his smile warmer. 'No, I just meant that you're a lovely, beautiful young woman and next time you're here I want to be able to see you smiling like you should be.' When he wrote out my prescription, he did so with the same flustered smile.

I was burning with anger and shame when I walked out, and I was even more angry that my mind had automatically made me feel about an inch high, when it wasn't me that should have been ashamed with myself. I told the receptionist what had happened and said that I wanted to book another session, and I did not want to see this doctor again. This was a man who saw himself as someone who treated illnesses, and so clearly, he didn't recognise depression as an illness. What a toxic attitude.

Part of me wanted to go back in and scream at the man. I wasn't here to cheat the system – I was doing everything I possibly could to get better and get into work as soon as possible. Not working was making me feel useless. Whereas most people woke up annoyed on a Monday morning because they had to go to work, I woke up every Monday feeling bad that I wasn't going to work. How dare he make feel stupid for that? Who the hell did he think he was?!

But in my experience, a message has never been heard through screaming. I hoped that what I said would make him think twice before saying something similar to anybody else, but that may have been naïve, wishful thinking.

Education doesn't happen overnight. It takes time to raise awareness, even for people who are supposed to help, and especially for people who are reluctant to learn about it or understand.

It wasn't all negative though. The other three doctors that I came across were much more supportive. One of them was understanding, but very matter-of-fact. Rather than make eye contact and talk through the topic in detail, he would type everything I said, and talked a lot about the medication and the dosage I was taking and how I was finding it. Clinical, yes, a bit impersonal, maybe, but still I was being taken seriously and being offered help.

Another was a young woman, perhaps the same age as me, still training to be a doctor. She took notes of the medication I was taking, and she asked about the physical side effects I was having. She asked my opinion: did I personally feel comfortable with the medication and the dosage she was prescribing? Did I feel that I needed any further support from her? How was finding a volunteering placement going? Did I still have enough support around me? What was new in my life since we last spoke? She would look directly at me when we spoke, she seemed interested, and she praised every little victory that I shared with her. She was fantastic.

Another lady was just as personally interested in my story. She lit up when I walked in the room, remembered my personal details, and enquired after my family. She asked how the driving lessons were going. I remember shedding real tears when looked me in the eye and told me that I was an inspiration, and that everything I had done to recover so far was something to be hugely proud of.

At that moment, I did feel proud; I would leave her office at the end of the session puffed up with pride, like a fluffy budgie.

CHAPTER 19

TOYS IN THE ATTIC

January 2016 arrived. Therapy took a break over Christmas, and in my first session of the new year, I discussed my goals with Peter. He asked me how I would like the therapy sessions to be guided over the next few weeks.

I told Peter that the talking, confiding, and venting that I had done in my first few months of therapy had been a massive help. That I felt some hope creeping back into my life. That I was starting to feel more able to cope with the strongest emotions.

However, I had now been unemployed for seven months and was starting to worry about the gap. I felt like a fragile feather floating along in the wind. I was moving, but I didn't feel like I had a lot of control over it. I felt as if something could happen at any time to come along and throw me off course.

I was happy that I was starting to improve, but I really didn't trust it. I was paranoid about the next thing that was going to go wrong. I felt that in order to go from just coping to progressing in life, I needed to have some tangible goals to drive me forward. Something that I could measure, something I couldn't doubt. Something to keep me busy until I felt ready to be working again. Perhaps something that would help push me towards working again. Something to give me pride, so that when I saw my friends and they told me about their new job / new home / new achievement, I wouldn't make myself feel so embarrassed or ashamed.

Should I set a weekly target? Peter felt that I shouldn't put too much pressure on myself, so we came to an agreement of a monthly goal. But holy hell! I had already spent the first few years of my twenties feeling like I was falling behind in life compared to all the people around me. And now this huge wobble had put me back another seven months. I was itching to get everything done quicker. To be better straightaway. To be cured right now. To fix everything, right this second.

So, I agreed to a monthly goal, but I admit that in my head I was already calculating what I would need to do to achieve each goal in two weeks instead.

'I have no idea what goal to choose first, though. It's like asking me to choose which pile of rubble to sift through and tidy first after an earthquake.'

Peter suggested I take a different approach. Instead of choosing a goal that I thought I should do, or that I thought others would expect of me, he asked me to visualise myself in four weeks' time, exactly where I wanted to be.

I told him that I couldn't stand the sight of my bedroom anymore. The old Disney Princess sheets that had originally been used whenever my nieces stayed over, the wardrobe full of clothes that my mother was storing for Lord knows how many members of the family, the bedside table from my old house, the blackout curtains that cut out the outside world while I tried to fall asleep through the tears. They were all horrible reminders of my breakdown and my difficult life before it. I needed to change it all. I felt as if I was leaving that chapter of my life behind me, so my surroundings needed to reflect that too.

I told Peter that I wanted a brand-new bedroom. A bedroom that reflected the creative, happy side of my personality that liked all things pretty. I wanted to care about every item that I owned, and I wanted everything in there to be something that brought me joy and pride when I looked at it. I wanted to shed the items that reminded me of a horrific time, or of the parts of my life that I was still grieving for. I wanted a brand-new space for a brand-new start. This was one of the first times after my breakdown that I knew I was genuinely ready to start looking forward, instead of looking back.

And so, we put together a list of the things that I could possibly do to make it happen. And then a determination was sparked within me. I had the time on my hands. I had supportive parents. What I didn't have was the money – I was still on sick pay. But that didn't put me off – in fact, I was going to prove just how thrifty I could be. Another way for me to be creative and crafty.

Now, I had always been a hoarder. I didn't like to throw things away. Whenever I did a 'spring clean' as a kid, I somehow managed to throw out what seemed like a lifetime's worth of things, while also clinging on to so many belongings that I'm surprised dragons hadn't set up home in the teetering towers of our treasures.

At this stage in my recovery, I had become addicted to Pinterest. I was pinning every article I could find about anxiety, depression, and recovery. I had stumbled across countless memes declaring 'Clutter is not just the stuff on your floor – it's anything that stands between you and the life you want to be living' (Peter Walsh), or 'Clutter is the physical manifestation of unmade decisions fuelled by procrastination' (Christina Scalise).

There were lots of articles circulating about things like the KonMari method of simplifying and organising the home. There were lots of variations upon the same, but the basic premise of all of them was this:

Items You Should Keep

1) You have used it in the last year.

2) You haven't used it in the last year, but only because it is seasonal or dependent on an occasion (e.g. a suitcase for holidays, a suit for weddings, a picnic basket for the summer).

3) It gives you joy to look at, or conveys memories / has sentimental meaning. Get it on display! But if it is in a box and you don't actually remember owning it until you have a spring clean, get rid of it.

4) You know exactly where it is in your house if you find yourself needing to use it.

5) You can't easily buy it at a local shop if you need it urgently. That's right. You don't need to keep hold of 50 pens. You can buy an emergency pack of 20 biros at the supermarket for a pound. We're in the digital age – when is the last time you so much as wrote a shopping list without an app?

It made so much sense. I realised that my clutter was a sign of my complete inability to move on from anything. And so I purged, on a massive scale.

In the space of a week, I went through every single worldly possession that I had. In my dad's house, the spare room was stacked, floor to ceiling, of with boxes of my belongings that Mam and Steph had moved out of my previous house for me. It was overwhelming to look at – a huge landscape of emotional rubble to sift through.

So, I took one box at a time, took it through to the next bedroom, and worked through the rubble, pebble by pebble. I didn't concentrate on the full project at hand. I didn't have 25 years of stuff to organise, I just had this box in front of me. One box. I could manage that.

I continued in this way. Soon, I had five boxes of items to sell, 12 bin bags of rubbish, and another 20 bin bags of stuff that went to the local charity shops. If I didn't absolutely need it, or it if it was something that could be replaced down the line, it went out the door. Some things I had kept for years and years, spring clean after spring clean. But I was ruthless. It was the most honest I had been with myself in a long time.

Step two: paperwork. I gathered every single paper, personal, legal, official or otherwise, and I spent the better part of a day filing it, sorting it, or shredding it into oblivion. I was still finding tiny bits of white confetti for a couple of weeks afterwards.

Step three: digital clutter. I went through my Kindle and I deleted every single book that I had never read, never finished, or realistically, was never going to read. I put all my photos into folders. I spent three hours in one sitting deleting thousands of emails and unsubscribing from hundreds of different websites that would otherwise have gone on sending me their newsletters forever. I was working towards that golden hallelujah moment of seeing 'inbox zero' pop onto the screen. I'll skip the harrowing moment when I realised that I could have simply copied and pasted each URL into a block list to send them all straight to my spam folder. After my eye stopped twitching, I told myself it was the ceremony of the whole laborious practice that actually mattered. And I'm sticking with that.

I went onto my phone and deleted every single text message I had stored. I reasoned that if there were messages from people with whom my relationship had changed, keeping their messages was not going to bring those relationships or friendships back. It was time to make new memories. It was time to practise moving on.

I went onto every website, online accoun, and forum that I could ever remember joining and deactivated, updated, or deleted my accounts.

It was absolutely one of the most cleansing, cathartic, and therapeutic things I have ever done. As a result, I felt a huge weight lift off my shoulders.

Endless opportunities for guilt (unused gifts). Gone.

Fear (*Have I missed any bill payments?*). Gone.

Social anxiety (*Oh my god, I haven't looked at my emails in months*). Gone.

Self-criticism (*I bought a bloody gym membership and I've not used it in forever*). Gone.

Grief (*We used to be so close, what on earth happened?*). Gone.

Stress (*I just can't get this place tidy, I was supposed to organise that cluttered bookcase forever ago, I'm useless*). Gone.

I knew exactly where I stood in my own life. Now, I knew every single item I owned. I knew what boxes they were in. I knew where to find them. I used them all often. I had space to put the things that I loved on display, and I had the space to store new things that I needed. I knew where I was financially. I had what was, essentially, a blank canvass.

The next mountain to tackle was creating a space for myself that I could feel happy and relaxed in – somewhere I could retreat to. In the bedroom, there were three pieces of 'furniture' that used to be kitchen cupboards. Before I had thrown my wobbly and come storming down to take over her house like a giant weeping toddler, my mother had been storing them in the spare bedroom. By the end of day one, I had stacked them to create a bookcase, painted them lemon yellow, and covered the shelves in a beautiful, floral, duck egg-

—

coloured fabric that my friend Victoria had bought for me. I painted a chest of drawers to match.

I had also unearthed two large notice boards, and a memory came back to me of being in Laura's room when we were teenagers. She had her own room which automatically meant I was incredibly jealous (I'd always shared one with my sisters). It was bright pink and green, and she had one huge cork board that spanned the length of one of the walls, all covered in posters, photographs, souvenirs and magazine pages. It was personality on display, proud and colourful. I had always wanted one.

The notice boards went up with Mam's help. I filled them with photographs of friends and family, inspirational postcards, party and wedding invitations and certificates, and my brother-in-law put up a giant mirror onto the next wall. I bought a floral armchair to sit and knit on, and Mam bought me a bonsai tree and a fluffy rug. I put out all my perfumes in a display and bought a jewellery stand. Dad came computer shopping with me and I bought myself the very PC that I find myself sitting at writing this book. He also treated me to brand-new bed covers that reminded me of Cath Kidston designs. And so, my girly, hay fever inducing floral bedroom – where I was going to rebuild my life – was born.

I felt brand-new.

Here is what I learned from that experience: things are just things. A book is just a book. A necklace is just a necklace. Whatever meaning those things hold for you is completely inside your head. Sometimes that's good, and sometimes that makes you happy. Sometimes the items become family heirlooms. Sometimes, though, it just isn't healthy. They cause a million and one emotions that clutter up your mind. But it is in your power to decide and dictate which way that goes.

Do yourself a favour. If you have a dress in your wardrobe that a family member bought for you and it never fit you, or wasn't your style, just donate it. Get it out of your wardrobe. Your family member won't remember it's there. It was two years ago, and you don't need that hit of guilt every single morning when you see it and shove more tops in front of it. That dress is still sitting there behind those tops, and that guilt is still sitting in your mind, even if you chose to ignore it. In a few months, you will have forgotten all about that dress, and you will be guilt-free when choosing what shirt to wear to the office. Someone out there could have found that dress in a used clothes shop and be wearing it every summer, feeling like a million dollars.

See that book you have on your bookshelf for that hobby that you never took up? It's okay to accept that you never learned Spanish, or you never learned to cook Thai cuisine, or you never learned how to play the guitar. You aren't admitting that you're a failure. You are just admitting that the time to learn those things just isn't now. Donate the book. Give it to a friend who is looking for a new hobby. If – and when – the time comes that you're inspired to try learning again, there will be a shop out there with a thousand books on how to learn. Getting rid of it now does not stop you revisiting it in the future. Clear your bookshelf. Sell some things, and use the money to go on a trip you've always wanted to do. Get rid of the self-criticism and stop mourning the person that you haven't become yet. There is plenty of time.

CHAPTER 20

GOOD ADVICES

I think I mentioned before in this book that when I was looking for a book to help me recover, I wanted one that gave me some real tips I could action to help get better quicker. So, I've summed up a handful of my recovery techniques here for you.

Tell Someone

I often wonder if my story would have gone differently if I had told someone from day one (whenever that was). Someone else may understand what is happening to you. Someone may be worried and it would make them relieved if you opened up to them. Either way. Please break the silence.

Find a Project

This was one of the best pieces of advice I can pass on from my therapist: get yourself a project. Personal, creative or fun, find a purpose where you can measure your achievements – it will give you something to get out of bed for. At the very least, it gives your mind a focus and a distraction from the things that are troubling you and helps promote mindfulness. Any achievements you make, big or small, go a long way to building up your shattered self-esteem.

It shouldn't be something you feel that you are obligated to do – nothing that would have negative consequences on your life if you don't finish it. If it involves anything with a deadline or expectations imposed by another person, then immediately there is pressure there, which is a disaster if you're feeling fragile. Set your own deadlines and your own goals. It gives you a sense of accomplishment when you have finished them but you aren't under any stress or answering to anyone if you don't meet them or have to amend them.

Everyone has something in them to give to the world. It can be something you create, manufacture, or fabricate, ending with something you can keep, display, gift, or put to good use. It can be something you learn, that you can use to educate or entertain the people around you, or to improve your professional prospects or meet new people.

I tried a fair few new hobbies. I took sewing classes. I tried to do some of my own furniture upcycling. I did lots of creative things – the funniest of which was when I tried origami with my friend Carly. A friend since the first year of college, Carly is hands down the most talented person I know – she can draw beautiful masterpieces and has mastered a million and one crafts that amaze me every time I see them. I own a Christmas card in which she has carved beautiful Christmas images. I own a jar with a below-the ocean-scene created by real sand, shells and fish made with beads. I have a painting of myself of my bedroom wall where I'm depicted in cartoon form with my arms full of knitting items. I even own a ukulele that she has beautifully painted to match my floral bedroom.

Carly brought the paper and the how-to-books to my house. I was going to be a creative genius too! I chose a daffodil. After a couple of hours, I had a hungover dandelion, but I had managed to forget my troubles for the couple of hours.

Me, I chose to learn to drive and to volunteer with my friend's start up business. Her creative small enterprise, Create Paradise, offered sewing classes amongst other things such as upcycling furniture, clothes-making and needle craft, all from a gorgeous vintage-style large house that served cakes to boot. I became the knitting and crochet teacher.

Take It Step by Step

Don't try to move a mountain. Focus on one small part at a time. You risk intimidation and overwhelm if you pressure yourself too much to everything Right Now. For example, do you want to go to a place that scares you? Start with just driving there, or jumping on the bus. Do that a few times, and when this isn't scary anymore, get out of the car. When this feels okay, stand at the doorway. Only go in when you are feeling confident with everything that comes before it. One step at a time. If you try to do everything at once, you may scare yourself into never attempting it again.

Spring Clean

Clear the clutter, and make a new start. Part ways with anything around you that is creating any bad feelings. Your home is somewhere you spend most of your time, and it makes a massive impact on your mood.

Therapy

There are many kinds. In this book, I fly the flag for EMDR, and it may work for you. But it is by far not the only choice. Have an assessment, and understand that it doesn't make you a failure or pathetic to need therapy. It is about maintaining your health, and shouldn't be seen as any different as going to the doctors or the dentist.

Read and Educate Yourself

Know what you're up against. You might be part of the way there by picking up a book like this one. Don't just use a web search – this can sometimes be as big a minefield as googling 'why do I have a stomach ache?' and finding you have a tumour the size of an alien inside you. Look for published works, find some support forums. Ask your therapist or doctor.

Get Back to Nature

Find somewhere green, away from the bustle of everyday life. Take a picnic, or listen to some music. Take photographs. It gives you distance from your situation and soothes anxiety.

Give Yourself a Break

Be kind to yourself. You matter. You're important, and finding happiness for yourself is okay. Speak to yourself the way you would speak to someone you love, because that's what you deserve. If somebody was walking around behind you all day every day, constantly telling you that you were rubbish, useless, a failure, ugly, or any of the million negative things you tell yourself, you would roundhouse kick them out of a window. Don't let the judge win.

Do Something That Makes Someone Else Happy

Depression is a lonesome disease. It makes you feel lonely while also isolating yourself. It's very self-focused and makes it hard to see anything beyond yourself. While you need to take every care of yourself you can, sometimes a great way to make yourself feel better is to make someone else happy, and removing the spotlight in your mind from yourself to someone you love, or even a needy stranger.

I am a genuine believer in the idea that if you have a positive view of someone, you should tell them. You never know what impact you will have. Even if people think you're that weirdo who compliments everyone, they'll still hear it.

In a society of negativity and low self-esteem like ours, people will hear everything you have to say about them. It will matter to them. Make it count, and let it be something encouraging, comforting, inspiring. Don't tear someone down to make yourself feel better, or make a point. We can all think of something that someone has said to hurt us that we still remember to this day, long after they have forgotten ever saying it. Make it something loving and complimentary, and a happy reaction will stay with you for a long time.

Challenge Your Negative Thoughts

One of the superpowers of that bitch we call anxiety is the ability to convince you that something you are imagining in your head is true. I can't believe the endless number of times that something I have been scared of has never come to pass. Just because you can picture something horribly in your mind – someone saying something horrible about you, something going horribly wrong – it doesn't make it true. You have to try to remind yourself that when we are anxious, we can see evidence of something we fear all around us. A certain thing that a person says or does could send us into a spiral of hurt and confusion because we're convinced that they've made a passive insult to us, meanwhile someone else could be feeling that it was about them.

In order to keep recovering from my obsessive rumination, a big part of what I tried to do when healing was making peace with my past. This is what EMDR was about of course, but for me it wasn't the only way of tackling it.

It's human nature to be threatened by something you don't understand. If someone does something strange, or somehow lives their lives differently to you, subconsciously you take it as a criticism. Why isn't that person living like you? Are they not 'normal?' Are you not 'normal'? Is there something wrong with the way you live your life if they are not choosing to live theirs in the same way?

In my experience, that's where a lot of animosity and jealousy and prejudice in this world comes from. Fear, and a lack of willingness to accept that something different from you isn't wrong, and that it isn't a criticism about yourself. It is a lot easier to write someone off as wrong, than to accept that there are people choosing to lead a different kind of lifestyle to your own. The most well-adjusted people I ever met in my life are those who feel completely at ease and confident enough in their own choices to accept, love and welcome others and all their differences.

If you can't make sense of it, it's much easier to make snap judgements and come to your own conclusions: a teen that is flying off the rails is just a demon child who wants to wreck their parents' lives. They're selfish and lazy and don't care about anybody else but themselves. They love the chaos they cause and they just want to hurt everyone around them.

You hate them. You call them every name under the sun. You have a bitter, sour feeling in the pit of your stomach when you think about it.

But what if that teen is struggling with a dark secret? What if they have been hurt by someone and nobody knows about it? What if they are filled to the brim with emotions that are so hard to bear that there just has to be an outlet? Could it hurt you less to try to connect with them and find out the real, raw, human reasons for doing the things they do?

Will I ever be able to apply this reasoning to the kids who bullied me? I don't know. Maybe it's something that will come to me long-term, maybe it won't. The fact is, I'll never know which of those kids were sadistic and cruel, and which were dealing with their own problems. It's not easy to make yourself forgive someone who might not deserve it – after all, I was miserable, but I didn't go out and beat anyone else up to make myself feel better.

I can't do anything now to change my feelings towards them. I think that ship has sailed. But, I can make a decision to think about situations in different ways going forward. No, it isn't easy. But it can be really freeing. I was able to forgive more, and a lot of hatred and anger disappeared. In turn, I had fewer dark, damaging feelings trapped inside me.

And so, what do we gain from this?

Hatred is tiring; it takes energy and it can be exhausting. But, still, hatred is so much easier than taking the time and patience to see another person's point of view. But at the end of the day, that person could be walking around out there, living their lives, and not thinking about you or your hatred. Their lives aren't affected by it. Hell, they may not even know how much you hate them to begin with.

The truth is, anger is not a nice feeling to carry around. It's even worse when it is directed at someone you are supposed to love, or someone who is a big part of your life. And anger and hate aren't solitary emotions. Most of the time, they come hand-in-hand with their best friends, hurt and betrayal. If somebody who had wronged me meant nothing to me, then I couldn't muster up the energy to hate them. They would be insignificant to me, not worth thinking about. We can believe that it feels satisfying, and that it can feel therapeutic to put energy into hating someone that has hurt you. But you aren't satisfied. You don't feel good. You're hurting. Making peace with your past doesn't mean that you will become a pushover, but it may just help you heal.

CHAPTER 21

FINEST WORKSONG

Even when you consider yourself to be recovered from depression, it can still pose a problem in different areas of your life.

When I had first approached the job centre at the beginning of my breakdown, I had received a medical note from the doctor to say that I wasn't in a state to be able to work. During one of the meetings to assess the validity of my application, I met a lovely woman who was very supportive when I told her that I was really motivated to get better so that I could work as soon as possible. She listened to the nature of the problems I was having and suggested a placement with an organisation called the Shaw Trust. She explained that the Shaw Trust was a charity in the UK, founded with the aim of getting people with disabilities and other disadvantages back into the workplace and becoming self-sufficient.

The Shaw Trust would provide me with my own mentor who would catch up with me on a regular basis to see how my recovery was going, and get to know me over the space of a few weeks to find out what kind of role would suit me best. She would also sign me up for workshops or similar opportunities that we both felt would help rebuild my confidence and help me network. I agreed straightaway – I didn't want to waste time, and if this place could help me get to a place where I could feel well enough to start applying for jobs, all the better.

I enjoyed the Shaw Trust. My mentor was a lot like me in personality, and I found her really easy to talk to. She understood what I wanted and what was worrying me. She knew when to encourage me to try the next step, whether it be mock interviews, or overhauling my CV, but she also knew when to reel me in when I started to panic that I was taking too long. For the sake of my own recovery she wanted me to avoid putting too much pressure on myself and doing everything too quickly.

I also signed up for sessions with a wellness mentor. He was interested in finding out my goals – professional and personal – and what my psychological barriers might be, so that we could work on removing them. I admired the way that he wanted to respect the therapy I was already having by making sure that anything we did together didn't clash with the course of treatment I was having with Peter.

In the Spring of 2016, after a two-week workshop that covered every aspect of job searching in depth – from CV writing to speculative letters to networking – we were required to take a mock interview. The Shaw Trust pulled out all the stops to make it as authentic as possible; I was to arrive at the 'interview' in full interview attire, and the Trust staff were to treat me as a stranger upon arrival. The whole interview was carried out as if I had never met the men conducting the session.

When I left the room after having shaken the hands of the two staff members and being assured that I would hear from them regarding the job within the week, I closed the door and heard cheering from the other side. I took that as good news, and when I received my official feedback the next day, I was ecstatic:

Terri has been an absolute pleasure to coach and at one time during our sessions, I handed the group over to her! She comes across as so confident, willing and able that I could honestly see her in a managerial role if she chose that route. She was always willing to support those members that weren't that confident and I thanked her for doing this.

I am sure that it was Terri that helped create such a good buzz and vibe within all the sessions; she is a natural leader. I did not see any of the issues that she mentioned in her barriers and I do hope that she has gone past this now and can focus on the future. I have every confidence that she will be successful with her job search, particularly when we look at how well she did at mock interview.

Terri's mock interview was by far the best I have ever taken part in while delivering these workshops. She scored a perfect ten in all of the answers she gave ... I could offer no recommendations to Terri other than to present in the same manner at a real interview and she will be successful! Enthusiasm and passion ooze from Terri in a natural fashion; she comes across as very likeable and genuine.

By the time I felt able to job search properly, I was really, really daunted by the concept, but it wasn't for the same reasons that I had been daunted when I was depressed – namely, that I had no talents left and had nothing to offer anyone. This time I was intimidated by the terrible state of the job market.

Aside from the odds being against me just based on pure numbers, I was now super aware of this glaring, empty gap on my CV. Yes, I had been keeping busy in the meantime – I was volunteering, learning to drive, taking up workshops at the Shaw Trust. But still, it was a gap in employment. They would want to know why I hadn't been hired in a year when I had a decent enough work and educational history.

The idea of trying to explain the gap to an employer in an interview was intimidating enough, but I worried about even getting to interview stage to begin with. The Shaw Trust had welcomed us to ask lots of questions – as many as we could think of – to help us improve our chances of landing a job we wanted. And I had one question that I asked over and over again.

'Should I mention the real reason that I was out of work for a year?'

The standard answer was quite straightforward. There was legislation in place that prevented employers from discriminating against you as a candidate on the basis of previous difficulties with mental health, especially if said problems would have no real bearing on the role for which you were applying. This was great, but in all honesty, it didn't ease my worries. Couldn't an employer just give any other made up reason for not hiring you? Couldn't they just *silently* discriminate against you if there was no evidence of them doing it? And what should I actually say to them? Should I avoid the word 'depression'?

I never really got a straight answer, but in all fairness, I don't think there is a correct answer. It's a sensitive topic, and the whole thing still has such a stigma around it. But knowing this didn't stop me worrying about it even more every time I wasn't offered a solution.

An opportunity for an experiment presented itself. An employer called me – it turned out it was for a job that I had applied for months ago when I had only just lost my job. It was in retail, and not really what I actually wanted to do. The interviewer's attitude on the phone stank so much that I was really glad I wasn't sitting in front of him. He asked me what salary I was looking at, and when I stated the salary that the job had been advertised at, he laughed patronisingly and said that he thought I was being a little over-optimistic.

The longer we spoke, the more I knew I wouldn't work for this guy with a gun to my head. So, when he asked the inevitable question – 'Why haven't you been employed for the last year?' I decided to go for it. I told him that I had been ill, and that I had taken the time to recover.

'Can I ask what illness you had?' I was fairly sure they weren't allowed to ask you that, but out of curiosity I answered his question. I told him that it had been depression, but that now I considered myself to be more than ready to get back into the workplace.

He paused. From what I could hear, he clicked his tongue and sucked his teeth. 'Hmmmm, right. And in what way would you say that would impact your role with us?'

Summoning up the spirit of teenage Terri, I gathered up as much sarcasm as I could muster in one breath.

'It won't impact the role. As I have *previously stated*, I took the time to make sure that I got myself back to full health.'

The interviewer sniffed, gave a few more obnoxious sighs and 'hmmm's that made me want to slap him before he rang off. I didn't want the job, but I was still completely disheartened by the experience. It had confirmed all my worst fears about the whole situation.

The only thing I could do was hope that the answer would come to me at the right time, and try to tell myself that any employer that turned me down because I had struggled with my mental health wasn't somebody that I wanted to work for to begin with. That was all well and good, but it didn't leave me with a huge number of prospects.

The phone wasn't ringing. I would spend hours at any one given time on an application, never to hear another word about it. Every time I saw a job that I thought I would be perfect for, I tried my best not to get my hopes up. I don't know if you've ever tried to be both enthusiastic enough about a job to write a glowing, 'You're an idiot if you don't hire me' application *and* try to convince yourself that, if you hear nothing back it's not a big deal. But if you haven't, I'll tell you now – it's not bloody easy.

CHAPTER 22

THE ONE I LOVE

Instead of working, the summer passed in a mix of driving lessons, sunbathing in the garden, long walks with my dad (which were now enjoyable and fun), volunteering for Victoria and socialising.

The girls from the shop I used to work at and I went out most weekends. Along with my friend Beckie, another girl I used to work with who loves shoes, jewellery, make-up, and all things glamourous, I rediscovered the joys I had lost when I stopped wearing jewellery those years before. I loved showing up at her house with a whole closet worth of options to wear and meeting Katie for a night of cocktails and gossip. I felt like a normal 26-year-old woman without the weight of the world on her shoulders.

My friend Lewis was getting married, I had been asked to be bridesmaid. I was looking forward to the wedding more than I could say. It would be the night before my birthday and I couldn't think of a nicer way to see in my 26th than being with dressed up with all of my friends, watching someone I loved getting married, and then having a laugh and a drink and a dance. I had the most fun that I could remember having in such a long time. I was ridiculously happy for Lewis. I was also so happy just to realise that I was happy, that I felt I would burst with contentment.

I was still seeing Peter, but far more infrequently now. I felt stronger in myself and as though I'd recovered from my depression.

I was finally okay with the fact that my relationship hadn't worked out. I had spent the first six months blaming myself for the whole thing. I was completely depressed and hadn't had any self-esteem to speak of for years. Of *course* it was all my fault, I was useless and unlovable and the whole thing was my own doing ...

But, now I knew that wasn't true.

In the next few months, my opinion changed, but it was no healthier. Once the heartbreak started fading and I started to build up some more self-worth, the anger and resentment found their way in. I then blamed *him* for the whole thing. I had been ill. I was his girlfriend and he had given up. He had been cold and completely unfeeling ...

But that wasn't true either.

Here is the truth: we had both played a huge part in ending what we'd once had. Yes, I had depression, but over the years I had also learned to take every bad mood, every bit of paranoia, and every frustration I ever had in life and throw it his way. I spoke to him like crap, I took everything for granted. I pulled him into arguments constantly, baiting him into rows that he had no way of winning, because I was determined to be angry with him no matter what way he handled it. I made our life together hostile. In turn, he never shared his thoughts or feelings on anything. He never even tried. Nothing could possibly be fixed without honest communication.

We were young when we got together. We had a lot of happy times, and they will always be there. But we made all our mistakes with each other and learned all our lessons. Together, we wrote the manual *What Not to Do!*

I supposed that, if we could take those lessons and put them into making our future relationships work, then there was definitely a silver lining in there.

Sometime around the end of August or beginning of September 2016, he had met a nice girl and they had been seeing each other for a few weeks. In all honesty, I had already guessed. But still, when I got the text message and read through to the end, I took a deep breath and waited for the pain to come crashing in on top of me.

It didn't. I took another couple of deep breaths, and re-read it. No stab of pain to the heart, no overpowering grief headache. Almost a year to the day that my life had crumbled to bits, I was completely okay. Not only was I okay, I was ridiculously relieved. In the first few months after we had broken up I was dreading this day and how much it would hurt, but it didn't. It was a happy moment.

I wished him luck, and just asked that we could all get along and be respectful of each other. He agreed and I was glad. It was the best outcome I could have hoped for.

As for myself, I had been enjoying being single for a long while. I had nothing but time for myself, my own projects, and my own recovery. It was a time of constant learning about my past and planning for my suddenly limitless future.

I was starting to look at an old acquaintance in a whole new light ... A friend of my friends, at Laura's birthday in April 2016, we had both taken a seat opposite each other at one end of the long tables in a restaurant where we were celebrating. I didn't know a whole lot about him, actually. I knew through the grapevine that he had been doing a computer course, so I asked him how it was going. I asked what was happening with the band he was in with two of our mutual friends.

Simon didn't give a generic 'Yeah it's going well, how have you been?' answer. He answered at length. He explained, in detail, about a course he was studying. He spoke a lot, and he spoke with ease. He also spoke about how he had suffered with depression for a few years beforehand and how he was starting to feel a lot better. He talked about it in detail and even teared up a little. It fascinated me.

People just didn't do that in my experience.

I was happy. I was confident. I was Making Stuff Happen ... I decided to go for it.

CHAPTER 23

THESE DAYS

So where am I now? And, emotionally speaking, the big question … have I been living happily ever after?

I was offered the Assistant Manager job back at the shop that I used to work for. I turned it down. It wasn't personal. I loved every one of the staff members there and still saw them all the time. My own boyfriend worked there! I know that some people who cared about me would have wondered why I made the decision to turn down full-time work when I had been unemployed for so long. But I couldn't go backwards. Too much had happened to me since I left, and that chapter of my life was over. I had to move forward to the next one, even though at the time, I had no idea what that future was going to look like.

After a number of months spent applying non-stop for work – and trying to resist the disheartened feeling every time I woke to an empty email inbox every Monday morning – I finally came across an advertisement for a customer services administrator with one or more foreign languages, including French. The role seemed tailor-made for me.

I got sick of just firing off a CV and being ignored. I found the email address of a recruitment consultant at the company that had posted the ad, and I emailed her directly.

'I've only just sent my CV,' I wrote, 'but I want to email you to draw your attention to it. I'm made for this job and have been searching for it for months.'

It took an interview with the recruitment agency, an interview with a French-speaking lady in the company, an interview with the lady who managed the customer services department, a maths test, and an interview with the global customer services manager – but I got the job!

It was different this time around. Before, I had gone into every single job interview I had ever had with a big drum solo of self-doubt ringing in my ears, and a chorus of 'you're a useless sack of crap' playing behind it. I always knew that my answers were embarrassing and I felt like a fraud when I listed off my 'achievements'. In my mind, any jobs I'd managed to get had been complete flukes, and one day my bosses were going to realise that I actually wasn't all the things I said I was.

I actually enjoyed the interviews this time round. I know! It doesn't sound real does it? This really was different and I felt different in myself. And I didn't feel like I was lying once. I told them that I enjoyed meeting new people, and it wasn't exaggerated. There was no smoke and mirrors when I told them that I knew I could do the job. When I said that I could be an asset to the team, I did so without irony. I was worth something. I was talented. And I deserved the role. I meant every word.

This level of healthy self-esteem suited me well. The lady from the recruitment agency told me that I seemed self-confident and comfortable in my own skin: at ease and sure of what I had to say.

I started the job and instantly felt at home with the four women in my department. They made me laugh. They were kind. They learned alongside me, and did everything they could to teach me everything I wanted to know with real patience. They have become my friends very quickly.

Two months into the job, I took the money I had made and found myself a flat in the middle of the city centre. Laura, as an estate agent, came with me to view it and put her stamp of approval on it. Hull had been declared the City of Culture for 2017 and I wanted to be in the middle of it all. I didn't want to spend another minute of time on the edge of society, hiding with embarrassment and shame from everybody. I was going to get out there and live as much as I could.

Simon and I are still together. We have spent ten months planning future holidays, taking trips, spending lazy Sundays doing creative hobbies side-by-side, eating out at every restaurant in the city, or just wasting time watching films. I have spent ten months laughing every single day. Embarrassingly for some, but not for him, I knit for him, and he wears it. With pride. I'm teaching him how to cook, and one day the plan is for him to teach me the ukulele.

But recently, my mental health took a couple of steps backwards. My life was like spinning plates; my relationship and work were spinning happily but I wasn't as on top of everything in my life as I wanted to be, and my social life and home life were starting to slow down. I was getting forgetful and less organised. I hadn't wanted to admit to myself, so things started getting on top of me again.

My anxiety had started to creep back, and I could feel it. One night, going to sleep at 8.00pm for what felt like the 17th night in a row, the tears started. Some nights, it was complete and utter indulgent self-pity due to my anxiety. Some nights it was complete and utter frustration and anger with myself. There was literal pillow punching and mini-screams of anger. And the next morning, I'd finally open my eyes to the face that awaited me from the mirror. It was not me looking back. It couldn't be. I've seen bad plastic surgery leave people looking more attractive. My eyes were puffy, my skin was grey, my cheeks were red and sore, and my hair was sticking to my face.

You know it's going to be a rough day when your first words are 'Oh, Christ, what is that?'

But the pollen season was upon us here and I claimed hay fever to anyone who looked at me in shock the next day. I couldn't tell the truth. I had recovered. I had come back from the darkest place I had ever experienced in my entire life, and now the grey clouds were pushing up against the edges again. Could I be honest with my loved ones? Could I tell them that I thought it was happening again? Should I be embarrassed at the hypocrisy of writing a *book* about the things I learned through my recovery? What right did I have to write something that is supposed to be 'inspirational'?

I have drawn lots of parallels between weight loss and recovery from anxiety and depression. Both take a long time to happen; it takes a long time to come to terms with the fact that you have the problem to begin with. It takes even longer to work up the nerve to face it and find the best way to tackle it. And then there's the trial and error, the dashed hopes, the ups and downs. You have to completely overhaul your daily habits, and make a huge commitment over a long period of time.

You're about to go on a night out, and you put that dress on. You know – the lucky one that you bought for your last birthday that cost you half your rent and made you feel like Beyoncé's more attractive sister. Only, this time you feel distinctly more like a manatee than you were imagining when you were daydreaming at your desk earlier that day. So, the next morning you put some jeans on. They always fit like a glove, they'll make you feel better. But they feel much tighter than the last time you dragged them out of the back of your wardrobe. And the beautiful cycle of self-disgust starts again.

A few weeks and several denial pizzas later, you finally decide to do something about it. And you do. And this time it works. Over the next few months, you find a steel resolve and focus, and you get those pounds off. People at work start to notice; your friends start to compliment you. And on that next night out, you wear an even *better* dress and feel like a million dollars.

And then, you treat yourself to a bottle of wine, or a sugary cocktail or 15, because, hey! You're celebrating. And you've been *so good* for *such a long time* that you've well and truly earned it. After so long, you've finally reached your target, and you deserve to spend time revelling in the 'new you'.

Tomorrow you'll be right back to your fruit infused water and dry crackers.

Only ... you fancy a takeaway, and you go for it (but with low fat mayonnaise and a Diet Coke, since you're not a complete animal). You're nice and slim now, so you know you won't be judged if you're seen eating it – and besides, what difference is one takeaway going to make after all these months of salads?

And so on and so forth, round and round and round ...

It may take a few months or even a couple of years, but slowly, one by one, the old habits come back, and the pounds creep back on. You've stopped making sure that you drink two litres of water a day, you've stopped counting the calories, you've stopped grilling everything, and your gym membership card hasn't seen the light of day since ... how many months ago? That can't be right, can it? And holy crap, you remember that even then you were feeling proud about getting 'back into exercising.'

Ah, self-disgust! Where have you been, my clingy old friend?

The key lesson I have pulled from this comparison is this: I recovered last year, but I didn't stop being human. I didn't become perfect, because there is no such thing, and I didn't become invincible.

Perhaps most importantly of all, I didn't realise that my learning wasn't finished. Here is what I have recently learned about low-level anxiety. I noticed it in myself, and once I did, I started seeing it in people around me too. I hear it all the time. That philosophy of 'I'll be happy when...'

'I'll be happy when I've found the man of my dreams.'

'I'll be happy when I'm a size 10.'

'It'll be fine when I've found my dream job.'

This way of thinking is dangerous for two reasons. For one, it means that you aren't allowing yourself to be completely happy with anything less than your long-term goals. Often, when I talk to people about going on holiday, they say things like 'It's a six-hour flight, it's going to be crap, I just can't wait to land and start my holiday.'

What do I think? I say enjoy the flight! You can't get to that holiday destination without flying. It has to happen, so why not enjoy it? Have a nice meal, read a book. Play cards with your friends. Share a bottle of wine. Have a sing along.

Sure, the flight is no beach in the Bahamas, but it's time that you're with the people you love. It's time that you're not slaving away at work. It's your time. Enjoying the journey won't take away how great the holiday will be.

Don't tell yourself that you can only be truly happy when you've got that high salary, when you've bought your dream home, when you're married, when you've got that beach body. That's a lot of pressure to put on yourself. You are allowed to stop and appreciate the journey. These days are part of your life too, and if you don't take the time to enjoy them, that's a whole chunk of your life you're spending daydreaming. It's okay to be proud of where you are now, even if where you are now is on a plane instead of in the Bahamas.

The other reason that this is a dangerous mindset is that sometimes, That Time comes and the thing you've been waiting for actually happens. And it doesn't solve all of your problems. Life isn't ever easy. It still isn't going to be skipping-through-the-meadows, all-singing-all-dancing-all-the-time, just because you've made that achievement. Some parts of life will still be a challenge. For me, that time came when I finally got into a job where I could use my degree, when I had my very own place to live, and when I had total independence. I had found a relationship with someone who wanted the same things as me and talked even more than I did!

And so now I was going to be completely happy, wasn't I?

I could stop all the things I had done to recover because I did recover. So, I stopped working on my emotional health and wellbeing. I got complacent and I stopped all of it. Therapy went completely by the wayside. I never knitted. Volunteering fizzled out. I stopped my driving lessons. I stopped contacting friends. I stopped calling and visiting my family regularly. The diary entries dried up. I forgot myself, and Terri started to disappear in the earthquake once again.

I spent a good few weeks wondering if I could ever be happy in the long term, if I couldn't even escape depression when I had everything I had wanted for years. I indulged in the self-pity, and then, when I had my first anxiety attack in a long, long time, I heard the alarm bells go off and started giving myself a proper talking to. I could wallow, or I could fight my way out of the rubble. Pebble by pebble.

I understand now that honestly, happiness isn't completely dependent on your circumstances. You can't fight low self-esteem by fitting into a smaller size bikini – those insecurities will just manifest themselves somewhere else in your life, until you deal with them on the inside.

So, instead of continuing to criticise myself for it and keeping it a secret, here is what I did.

I arrived at the office at 7.30am. I opened the shutters. I got all the coffee cups ready, turned on my computer and did the usual reports for the girls. Unassuming Lena walked in with her usual beaming smile, and asked how I was coping with the hay fever that morning.

'Lena ... can I talk to you about something personal?' is all I managed to get out before my face did that oh-so-attractive crumply thing when I start to cry. 'I'm scared to talk to my family about it because I don't want to upset or worry them, and I've cut myself off from my friends, and I've felt too anxious to call any of them in weeks. But I need to get this out.'

Lena jumped up and headed straight for the box of tissues. 'Is there anything I can do to help?' Her natural instinct.

'I just need to let someone know. I know you all know I keep coming to work anywhere up to an hour-and-a-half before I'm supposed to start, and staying for just as long on an evening. I'm not sleeping properly, and, if I'm on my own at home, I'll eat and then go to sleep as early as half-past-seven, just to stop feeling stressed and down. I know why it's happening, I know what I need to do. I just need to say it out loud and make sure I'm not keeping it to myself, because keeping it as a secret is making it so much worse.'

Anne and Debbie came in shortly after. I repeated my explanation. I needed someone to know, I needed to have it off my chest and I needed to be able to speak about it without worrying that I was hurting someone. They instructed me to call Simon after work. They demanded that I always pick up the phone to tell them and vent whenever things were getting too much for me. Debbie made me a cup of tea and told me how loved I was, Anne shared a couple of tales of her own similar experiences, and they made me feel completely normal.

Then, when I left, I called Simon.

'Hey! How was work?'

So, I was blatantly honest. And I told him what I did. I was surprised at how level my voice was, and how matter-of-fact I sounded, and how I didn't apologise for it. I didn't tell him that I was useless or good-for-nothing. I told him I had an illness and was having a dip. I didn't say that I didn't know what to do and everything was going to be terrible. I told him what I needed to do, but just that I needed the help and support to do it. And I felt proud for it.

If he was taken aback to receive such a serious answer to such a casual question, he didn't come across that way. Neither was he stumped. He stayed calm and, actually, he did most of the talking. There wasn't a hint of judgement, disbelief, frustration or difficulty in understanding the problem. He saw it with perfect clarity. And he told me we would work on it together, in small steps so it wasn't overwhelming. And over the next couple of weeks, he kept those promises.

And here is what I am going to do, going forward. I have bought myself a new set of brightly coloured pens – the kind we use at work that are super-satisfyingly easily to write with. (I can't explain the level of sorrow I had when I went to the stationery cupboard at work and they had been replaced with generic scratchy ballpoints!) I am going to restart a diary. Tomorrow, I will purchase a few thousand minutes on my phone tariff and I will call all the people that mean the world to me, and tell them I want to hear their news. I'll write a list of the things I want to start doing again. I'll plan something social. I'll go back to therapy, and do some EMDR to help with the memories of the actual breakdown itself. I'll do it step by step.

I'll find Terri again, because I know she's still there, a lot closer to the surface than she was the last time I lost her.

To the reader who may be struggling with depression or anxiety, or both: you and I will have relapses. That's normal. But you won't be the same afterwards. You can't un-experience the things that have changed you. The next time something like this happens, you will come back slightly faster. You will recognise the warning signs sooner. And you must, in the words of my fantastic therapist, be kind to yourself, every single time – for the sake of yourself, and of the people who love you. Without self-compassion, you aren't free to heal.

It's August. It's raining lightly outside right now, but tomorrow it's supposed to be sunny. A shiny, happy day.

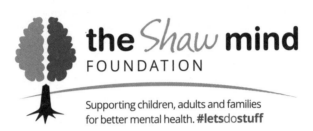

the Shaw mind

FOUNDATION

Supporting children, adults and families
for better mental health. **#letsdostuff**

Sign up to our charity, The Shaw Mind Foundation

www.shawmindfoundation.org

and keep in touch with us; we would love to hear from you.

We aim to bring to an end the suffering and despair caused
by mental health issues. Our goal is to make help and support
available for every single person in society, from all walks of life.
We will never stop offering hope. These are our promises.